CLINICAL COMPANION
FOR

ASSESSMENT
OF THE
OLDER ADULT

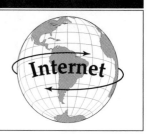

CLINICAL COMPANION
FOR

ASSESSMENT OF THE OLDER ADULT

Cora D. Zembrzuski, RN, MSN, CS, PhDc

New York University
New York, NY
and
The Connecticut Visiting Nurses' Association

DELMAR

THOMSON LEARNING   Australia Canada Mexico Singapore Spain United Kingdom United States

NOTICE TO THE READER

Publisher does not warrant or guarantee any of the products described herein or perform any independent analysis in connection with any of the product information contained herein. Publisher does not assume, and expressly disclaims, any obligation to obtain and include information other than that provided to it by the manufacturer.

The reader is expressly warned to consider and adopt all safety precautions that might be indicated by the activities herein and to avoid all potential hazards. By following the instructions contained herein, the reader willingly assumes all risks in connection with such instructions.

The publisher makes no representation or warranties of any kind, including but not limited to the warranties of fitness for particular purpose or merchantability, nor are any such representations implied with respect to the material set forth herein, and the publisher takes no responsibility with respect to such material. The publisher shall not be liable for any special, consequential, or exemplary damages resulting, in whole or part, from the readers' use of, or reliance upon, this material.

Delmar Staff
Business Unit Director: William Brottmiller
Executive Editor: Cathy L. Esperti
Acquisitions Editor: Matthew Kane
Developmental Editor: Patricia A. Gaworecki
Editorial Assistant: Shelley Esposito
Executive Marketing Manager: Dawn F. Gerrain
Channel Manager: Tara S. Carter
Executive Production Manager: Karen Leet
Project Editor: Pat Gillvan
Production Coordinator: Nina Lontrato
Art/Design Coordinator: Jay Purcell

Delmar Publishers
3 Columbia Circle
Box 15015
Albany, New York
12212-5015

International Thomson
Publishing Europe
Berkshire House 168-173
High Holborn
London, WC1V 7AA
England

Thomas Nelson Australia
102 Dodds Street
South Melbourne, 3205
Victoria, Australia

Nelson Canada
1120 Birchmont Road
Scarborough, Ontario
Canada, M1K 5G4

International Thomson
Editores
Campos Eliseos 385
Piso 7
Col Polanco
11560 Mexico DF Mexico

International Thomson
Publishing GmbH
Konigswinterer Strasse 418
53227 Bonn
Germany

International Thomson
Publishing Asia
221 Henderson Road
#05-10 Henderson Building
Singapore 0315

International Thomson
Publishing—Japan
Hirakawacho Kyowa
Building, 3F
2-2-1 Hirakawacho
Chiyoda-ku, Tokyo 102
Japan

ISBN: 0766807304

Dedication

To Mark, David, and Sara, for their love and sense of humor; to my mother, Lucy, who instilled the value of creativity in me; to Suzi, my "sister" for her eternal support; to Cheryl O., friend, organizer, and typist; to the patience and never-ending kindness of Patty, my editor.

And to all those nursing students and nurses around the globe who advocate and care for older people every day.

Contents

Preface

There is global interest in older people—who they are, their characteristics, how are they alike and dissimilar from other age groups and, especially, how they age. Clinicians refer to "abnormal" and "normal" aging, yet segments of the research conducted was on older people with diseases. Currently, the distinctions between normal and abnormal are becoming less clear as "baby boomers" become targets of inquiry as they age, the lines of distinction will become even fuzzier. The intention of the *Clinical Companion for the Assessment of the Older Adult* is to provide a convenient and succinct reference to physical, psychosocial, spiritual and cultural dimensions of care for the older client. That it can be tucked into the pocket of a labcoat makes it a convenient reference book in any clinical setting where students as well as practicing nurses and clinicians are providing care to the older population.

Conceptual Approach

The companion is not a cookbook; it utilizes a scientific body systems approach along with sensitivity to the assessment of older people. Traditional physical assessment skills are incorporated with age-related changes, as we currently understand them. The over-arching focus gently integrated into the clinical companion is that of prevention and health teaching, interdisciplinary team care, and quality of life of the older adult; these are integral to holistic and effective nursing care in such a complex population. Moreover, the *Clinical Companion for the Assessment of the Older Adult* reflects the complexities in the older population, which mandate a broader examination and a more expansive approach to assessment and care.

In addition, the clinical companion may be used in conjunction with the core text by Mildred Hogstel, *Gerontology: Nursing Care of the Older Adult,* or alone.

Organization

The companion is comprised of 16 chapters divided by physiological systems while presenting special assessments used frequently in the older population. There are ten appendices that provide special assessment instruments such as the Mini Mental State Exam, summary of AHCPR guidelines for pressure ulcer assessment, pain assessment, and laboratory values in older adults. A full glossary that includes definitions of all the Key Terms is included at the end of the book.

Special Features

- Key Terms are listed at the beginning of each chapter and boldfaced in the chapter text. Key terms comprise the glossary at the end of the book.
- Tips From the Experts opens each chapter with a relevant tip, procedure guideline or best practice from experienced practitioners with the older adult population.
- Nursing Checklists offer an organizational framework for the assessment process or for approaching certain tasks.
- Nursing Tips help the reader apply basic knowledge to real life situations and offer useful hints and shortcuts when working with the older client.
- Nursing Alert highlights potentially serious or life-threatening signs or critical assessment findings that require immediate action to ensure the safety of the client.

Reviewers

Marilyn J. Vontz, PhD, RN, MSN, MA, BS
Professor
Bryan Hospital School of Nursing
Lincoln, Nebraska

Ada Romaine Davis, PhD, RN, CANP
Professor Emeritus
Johns Hopkins University
Baltimore, Maryland

The Nursing Process, the Older Adult, and the Nurse

Key Terms

assessment
evaluation
implementation
intervention
mutual goal-setting
nursing diagnosis
outcome
planning

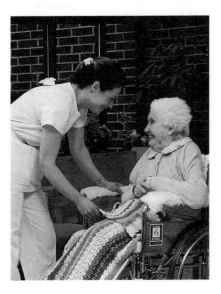

TIPS FROM THE EXPERTS

1. Plan several assessment sessions. Most older adults do not wish or are not able to tolerate lengthy sessions.
2. Tend to details on all aspects of the nursing process; take the time up front.
3. Don't skip steps; quick conclusions usually result in errors.
4. Listen carefully and allow the older person to speak for herself or himself; show respect for the family, but do not assume that the older persons' family *always* knows best.
5. Be a team player; collaborate with other disciplines to provide the best possible care for the older person.

Although there are many theories and approaches to nursing, the nursing process is the most widely accepted way in which most nurses practice nursing, as an art and science, in most settings. Nursing theories and views on nursing practice focus on the nature of humans, their environment, and the meaning of health (Fawcett, 1995). It is through this special lens that nurses care for people across the life span. What makes caring for older people different than caring for middle-aged adults or infants? There are certainly commonalities—we are all human! There are also distinctions that make life at 80 equally as unique an experience as life at 39.

The following five sections examine and discuss the nursing process relative to older people, distinguishing some of their unique qualities. It is important to note the overarching framework of interdisciplinary care paramount to nursing practice, which successfully approaches the complexities posed by older people. More simply, nursing does not and cannot be practiced in isolation from other disciplines while promoting effective care for older people. Coordination of care and the teamwork of *all* disciplines are required to promote and maintain the best possible health and environment for older people.

Assessment

The basic dictionary meaning of *assess* means to assign value to something, to calculate, to consider, and to estimate. Assessment is an estimation or account of something. To assess, in nursing, means to make sense of what one observes. In this regard, assessment is the foundation of compiled observations and data, subjectively from the client's viewpoint, objectively and intuitively from the nurse's viewpoint. Assessment of older adults can appear overwhelming, given the many years of experience and health history that they encompass. It is challenging to sort out what might be significant or insignificant from the health history. While guided interview questions are essential to a systematic approach to collecting data, allowing plenty of time to capture the richness of information is equally compelling. If the assessment process is shortchanged, there is a danger of inaccurate, missing, or incomplete data on which to base care. It is wise, if possible, to plan several sessions for obtaining the health history and physical examination. In addition, physician, social worker, case manager, physical therapist, and other key health care team members will want to interview the client to obtain essential information on past history, current status, and related self-care and interpersonal issues.

Health History

The health history is an important cornerstone of assessment data on the older person. As an older person reveals subjective perception and viewpoint, he or she conveys thoughts, feelings, and deep-rooted individual attitudes influencing health. Not all aspects of the health history are verifiable. For example, if the individual states she had a hysterectomy in 1959 and "from then on, suffered from depression for years to come," verification of the date is not as important as pursuing the line of questioning about the depression. By the end of the health history, the nurse will be able to determine potential themes, issues, and hunches pertinent to care. Other valuable sources of health history include family members, friends, and previous medical records. Nevertheless, the individual is the prime source; even when mild memory or cognitive deficits are present, the individual's attitude, outlook, and general valuation of life are gleaned from interacting directly with the older person. (Chapter 3 offers a more comprehensive account of the health history.)

Physical Assessment

Physical assessment is best described as the set of objective facts and findings obtained through the clinician's skills of observation (looking), listening (ausculation and percussion), feeling (palpating), and intuiting (sensing). In addition, common measurements such as blood pressure, glucose monitoring and results of laboratory tests, tests of memory, cognition, and depression, as well as functional assessment measures are employed in order to understand the person's baseline status in these areas. Although many older people have numerous and similar medical diagnoses (comorbidities), their baseline status and capacity to maintain a positive quality of life vary. For example, many older people may share the diagnosis of congestive heart failure, yet their abilities to cook, clean, go to the movies, and enjoy life may be dramatically different. Concrete assessment parameters are useful in measuring the degree to which the individual compares with a norm. As a result, abnormal findings, although not conclusive in themselves, prompt further investigation and assessment by other members of the health care team. A modified body system approach paired with specialized tests is useful in contributing to care planning and preventive care.

Nursing Diagnosis

Nursing diagnoses, unlike medical diagnoses, are based on the ways in which humans respond to illnesses. Problems are identified as active or potential. Acute, chronic, preventive, and maintenance issues are addressed through the taxonomy of the North American Nursing Diagnosis (NANDA) classification. After all assessment data is completed, the nurse critically examines and synthesizes the meaning and implications of the information. Keen judgment and the ability to step back and synthesize the wide array of information presented about the older person results in arriving at priority areas of care. Through use of nursing diagnoses, there is uniformity in categorizing the individual's needs. Some settings do not use nursing diagnoses; instead, the older person's needs and problems are clearly identified and described. Refer to the Appendix for a current list of nursing diagnoses.

Table 1-1 lists some nursing diagnoses associated with problems, risks, or potential problems experienced by older people. The table combines common issues and body systems targeted for assessment. The table is intended to be a quick reference.

Planning

The planning phase of the nursing process involves closer examination of nursing diagnoses, **mutual goal-setting** with the older person, and establishment of nursing **interventions** or approaches to facilitate client **outcomes.** Prioritization is essential when planning care. In most instances, physiological needs take priority. Examples of basic physiological needs are need for sleep, comfort (pain-free), food, and water. Because many older adults have multiple and complex needs, the nurse will uncover numerous nursing diagnoses. These diagnoses are then prioritized according to importance. Maslow's Hierarchy of Needs (Figure 1-1) is a common framework used to sort out and direct the sequence of resolving client care problems.

Goals are broad and somewhat general statements. Goals are formulated with the older person. In addition, outcomes are established. Outcomes are statements of desired changes in client behavior. An example of a goal is, "The client will ambulate throughout his home." The outcome is, "The client will be able to walk 20 feet three times/day by June 30." Note that the outcome is specific, is measurable, has a time frame, and supports the goal.

Goals and outcomes generate interventions. Interventions are specific and scientifically based actions and strategies used by the nurse and the interdisciplinary team to promote goal accomplishment and positive client outcomes. Two examples are, "The nurse and dietitian will spend one-half hour/day reviewing information on the low-sodium diet," or "The nurse will demonstrate drawing up the client's insulin and view two return demonstrations." Similar to outcomes, the health care team's interventions are highly specific and directed. The team and each individual member are accountable and

Table 1-1   Issues/Body Systems and Nursing Diagnoses Common to Older People

Pattern 1 = Exchanging
Pattern 2 = Communicating
Pattern 3 = Relating
Pattern 4 = Valuing
Pattern 5 = Choosing

Pattern 6 = Moving
Pattern 7 = Perceiving
Pattern 8 = Knowing
Pattern 9 = Feeling

ISSUES/ BODY SYSTEMS	PATTERN	RELATED NURSING DIAGNOSES
Skin, hair, and nails	1	• Impaired skin integrity • Impaired tissue integrity
Head and neck	1	• Decreased adaptive capacity: intracranial
Sensory: eyes, ears, nose, throat, mouth	7	• Sensory/perceptual alterations (specify visual, auditory, kinesthetic, gustatory, tactile, olfactory)
	1	• Altered dentition • Altered oral mucous membranes
	6	• Risk for suffocation • Impaired swallowing
Respiratory	1	• Impaired gas exchange • Ineffective airway clearance • Ineffective breathing pattern
Cardiovascular	1	• Decreased cardiac output • Altered tissue perfusion, cardiopulmonary
Breasts and nodes	7 8	• Body image disturbance • Knowledge deficit, breast self-examination
Musculoskeletal and functional	6	• Impaired physical mobility • Impaired wheelchair mobility • Activity intolerance • Fatigue • Self-care deficit (specify)
	1	• Risk for injury • Risk for disuse syndrome
Neurological	9 1	• Chronic pain • Dysreflexia • Energy field disturbance
	8	• Chronic confusion • Acute confusion
Mental health	9	• Anxiety • Fear
	5	• Ineffective individual coping • Noncompliance (specify) • Ineffective management of therapeutic regimen

continued

ISSUES/ BODY SYSTEMS	PATTERN	RELATED NURSING DIAGNOSES
	2	• Impaired verbal communication
	5	• Decisional conflict (specify)
	8	• Altered thought processes
		• Impaired memory
Psychosocial well-being	6	• Adult failure to thrive
	3	• Altered role performance
		• Social isolation
		• Risk for loneliness
		• Impaired social interaction
		• Caregiver role strain
	5	• Health-seeking behaviors
	7	• Chronic sorrow
		• Hopelessness
		• Powerlessness
Nutritional	1	• Altered nutrition, less than or more than body requirements
		• Fluid volume excess
		• Fluid volume deficit
Abdominal	1	• Bowel incontinence
		• Constipation
		• Diarrhea
		• Altered urinary elimination
		• Urinary incontinence (separate diagnoses: stress, urge, functional, reflex)
		• Urinary retention
Male and female genitalia	3	• Sexual dysfunction
		• Altered sexuality patterns
Endocrine and immune	6	• Delayed surgical recovery
	1	• Risk for infection
		• Ineffective thermoregulation
		• Risk for altered body temperature
		• Hypothermia
		• Hyperthermia
		• Altered protection
Spirituality	4	• Spiritual distress
		• Potential for enhanced spiritual well-being

Nursing diagnoses from *NANDA Nursing Diagnoses: Definitions and Classification 1999–2001*, by NANDA, 1998, Philadelphia: Author.

responsible for actions and contributions toward meeting the client's goals.

Implementation

The fourth phase, implementation, requires carrying out the nursing interventions, coordinating the health care team, and monitoring the health care team's progress. Implementation is "fluid," that is, if strategies are found to be not working, changes are made accordingly. For example, while teaching a client about his low-sodium diet, he experiences angina. The

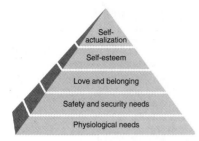

Figure 1-1   Maslow's Hierarchy of Needs

NURSING CHECKLIST

Nursing Process

A = assessment of client's health needs
D = analyze, diagnose, and prioritize from assessment findings
P = plan mutually agreeable outcomes and interventions
I = implement actions along with the interdisciplinary team
E = evaluate the client's progress on outcomes
R = reassess and readjust toward maximum outcomes

---

teaching must be postponed and rescheduled. Consequently, the goal may take longer to achieve than what was initially anticipated. This is a common occurrence in implementation and warrants the flexibility and patience of the nurse and the health care team without losing sight of the client outcome.

Evaluation

Evaluation, the final step in the nursing process, requires clinical judgment. Several questions need to be examined. Were outcomes achieved and were the goals accomplished? If no, why not, and what can be done to enhance goal accomplishment? If yes, how can the client build on these goals?

Evaluation of outcomes ought not to occur at the end of the time frame designated for goal achievement. For example, take the case of weight loss—"alteration in nutrition, less than body requirement." If the nurse ignores weekly or daily monitoring of weight, potentially the weight loss may progress to dangerous levels. Thus, evaluation of the older person's progress in accomplishing goals is paramount to preventing life-threatening problems, complications, or negative outcomes.

In addition, the nurse should seek feedback to find out whether the older person feels that health care outcomes and goals were successfully achieved. Sometimes positive outcomes are attained but at personal costs. Again, take the case of progressive negative weight loss. A client may have achieved the outcome of gaining 4 pounds in a month. However, she may tell the nurse that she hates the liquid dietary supplement. As a result, other options such as "natural" foods—fruits and yogurt—become necessary to enhance pleasure in eating and quality of life. Be mindful that the nursing process does not stop at evaluation. The process is dynamic and cyclical and feeds back into assessment.

The nurse's knowledge of health care, its systems, processes, and complexities, and of gerontology often situate her in the role of coordinator of care. The nurse is in a position to advocate for the needs of the older person and convey, as a spokesperson if necessary, the wishes of the client in a nonpatronizing manner. Together, nurse and client pave the way to health as the client wishes it to be. Realistically, not *all* individuals are motivated to follow *all* recommendations for "healthy living"; they select the aspects and standards of "healthy living" that *reasonably* fit into their lifestyle given who they are—likes and dislikes, limits and desires. The older person's individuality and preferences warrant respect and a nonjudgmental stance by all health care members.

Summary

There are five phases of the nursing process: assessment, diagnosis, planning, implementation, and evaluation. The process is cyclical and ongoing, and requires prioritization of needs. Given the rich history and complexity of older adults, the nurse must take the time to observe, tend to detail, synthesize, and coordinate care with the client, the family, and the interdisciplinary health care team. Quality of life and the older person's wishes are primary considerations when carrying out the nursing process.

References

Fawcett, J. (1995). *Analysis and evaluation of conceptual models of nursing* (3rd ed.). Philadelphia: F. A. Davis Company.

North American Nursing Diagnosis Association (NANDA). 1998. *NANDA nursing diagnoses: Definitions & classification 1999–2001.* Philadelphia: Author.

2

Physical Assessment Components

Key Terms

auscultation
inspection
palpation
percussion

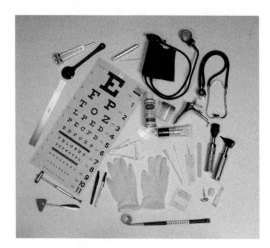

The physical examination uses techniques of inspection, palpation, percussion, and auscultation. By far, inspection is the most frequently used skill; much is gleaned from paying attention to what is observed. Physical assessment obtains and analyzes the data from the comprehensive health history and the physical examination. The tools of assessment are introduced in this chapter, with special focus on older persons.

Aspects of Physical Assessment

The purpose of physical assessment in an older person is fourfold:

1. to provide baseline data to gauge changes in condition and health status
2. to validate the health history and investigate current complaints
3. to prevent recurrent and debilitating problems
4. to support the plan of care

Depending on point of entry into the health care system, physical assessment may occur:

- in an emergency
- periodically by a primary care provider
- on a small scale to investigate a complaint
- as required by regulatory entities in the nursing home and in home care
- not at all because of lack of accessibility to the health care system

Role of the Gerontological Nurse

The role of the gerontological nurse combines expert knowledge on aging and pathology in older people with sensitivity to their innermost concerns. It is not common during a physical examination to hear, "Why do you waste your time on me?" or "Do you really think you can help me? I'm too old!" It is important to stop,

look, and listen to the meaning of what is said. As assessment unfolds, so will recurrent themes and persistent messages from which needs are identified.

As mentioned previously, the gerontological nurse often takes on a leadership and advocacy role in guiding and coordinating appropriate care in a specific setting during episodic or chronic illness. It is evident that the nurse stands side by side with the client, clinically and ethically. To this end, a unique bond is formed between the older person and the gerontological nurse that evokes trust and security.

Standard Precautions

Standard (universal) precautions are maintained during physical examination to protect the client and the nurse from infectious diseases. If contact, splashing, or soiling by body fluids is anticipated, gloves, gown, mask, and/or goggles are donned.

Basic to preventing the spread of infection is good handwashing. This has been drilled into most of us in nursing school and throughout our careers. Handwashing protects both you and your client. Generally, older people have greater difficulty fighting off and healing from infections; it is thus very important to think preventively. Follow Center for Disease Control Guidelines, which are readily available at your place of employment or on the CDC web page.

⚡ NURSING ALERT

Do you know if you or your client has a latex allergy? Many gloves are made from latex. Find out if your client is allergic to latex before using latex gloves in the examination. Symptoms range from dermatitis to anaphylactic shock.

Assessment Techniques

The four techniques that provide objective assessment data are inspection, palpation, percussion, and auscultation. A less tangible step—intuiting or sensing—combines all four techniques.

Inspection

To inspect means to see something with a "discerning eye." Relative to the assessment process, inspection requires the use of visual and olfactory senses. The process of inspection begins upon meeting the client. Posture and stance, balance, walking, and eye contact are all aspects of inspection. The gerontological nurse makes sense of what is seen/smelled based on a specific framework—that of gerontological nursing. For example, how an older person walks is critical to her or his ability to negotiate movement throughout her or his environment/household. How the person carries himself or herself also has potential implications for the older person's self-esteem, self-care, physiological well-being, and psychosocial well-being. Hygiene and health issues will surface and may be noted through particular odors, although odors alone are not conclusive evidence of problems—they are clues and prompts for further investigation. Inspection requires adequate lighting and the nurse's attentiveness.

Palpation

Palpation requires warm hands and a gentle touch. Deep palpation is not used nearly as often as light palpation in older people. As with any procedure, explain to the client where you will be pressing and why. No one appreciates surprises. Our hands are extensions of expression and caring. They should be used as therapeutic tools to convey respect and concern for well-being. Clients know when hands convey a rough touch or are hurried. Again, take the time to convey care and respect despite a busy schedule.

Different parts of the hand are best used for different types of palpation. Finger pads are used most frequently to feel for body organs—placement, size, shape, mobility, and masses. The dorsum or back of the hand is best used to discern body temperature, whereas the palmar or ulnar surface (fingers and palms) are best able to pick up vibrations. Light and deep palpation will be described, although light palpation is used most often in the assessment of older people.

Light Palpation

Light palpation requires:

- Gentle use of finger pads
- Depressed approximately 1 cm
- To discern obvious masses and abnormalities, skin texture, and moisture and tenderness

Refer to Figure 2-1.

Note that the finger pads are kept together. The motion is circular, not lifting from the area but moving adjacently from section to section. Clients will comment that palpation feels like massage. However, the purpose of massage and palpation is much different and should be explained to the client.

Deep Palpation

Deep palpation is used in the following ways:

- Finger pads are used
- Depressed approximately 4–5 cm
- Used most frequently in abdominal assessment
- Shape of masses and their mobility are identified

Refer to Figure 2-2 and Chapter 15 on deep palpation in abdominal assessment.

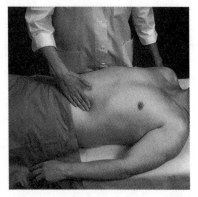

Figure 2-1 Technique of Light Palpation

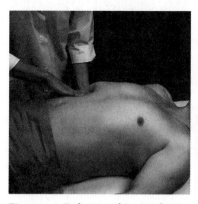

Figure 2-2 Technique of Deep Palpation

Percussion

Percussion requires tapping motions to distinguish degrees of fullness and density. Air, solids, and fluids create distinctive sounds, which connote normal or abnormal findings. Characteristics of percussion sounds are shown in Table 2-1.

The types of sounds include:

- Flatness
- Dullness
- Resonance
- Hyperresonance
- Tympany

Intensity, duration, and pitch are also analyzed (see Table 2-1). It is important to note that the denser the substance, the higher the pitch; also air-filled structures are louder and lower-pitched than structures containing less air. Think of the emphysematic lung as a hollow drum and very loud and low-pitched whereas the intestines holding air pockets will be tympanic and high-pitched. Practice percussion on friends and colleagues. Immediate (direct) and mediate (indirect) percussion is used to ascertain sounds from particular body densities. Direct fist and indirect fist percussion will be illustrated although this is rarely used on older persons. Immediate percussion (Figure 2-3) is used especially on sinuses. It requires direct tapping on the sinuses.

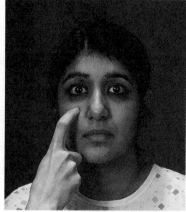

Figure 2-3 Technique of Immediate Percussion

Mediate (indirect) percussion (Figure 2-4) requires the following:

- Nondominant hand is placed on the surface
- Middle finger is extended on exact location
- Clear the middle finger by fanning the remaining fingers outward
- With dominant hand, use the middle finger to strike between the distal interphalangeal point and the finger-

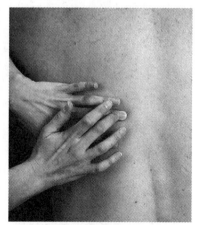

Figure 2-4   Technique of Mediate Percussion

Table 2-1 Characteristics of Percussion Sounds

SOUND	INTENSITY	DURATION	PITCH	QUALITY	NORMAL LOCATION	ABNORMAL LOCATION	DENSITY
Flatness	Soft	Short	High	Flat	Muscle (thigh) or bone	Lungs (severe pneumonia)	Most dense
Dullness	Moderate	Moderate	High	Thud	Organs (liver)	Lungs (atelectasis)	
Resonance	Loud	Moderate-long	Low	Hollow	Normal lungs	No abnormal location	↓
Hyperresonance	Very loud	Long	Very low	Boom	No normal location	Lungs (emphysema)	
Tympany	Loud	Long	High	Drum	Gastric air bubble	Lungs (large pneumothorax)	Least dense

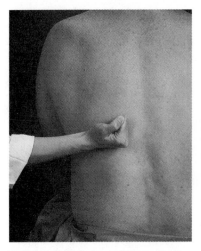

Figure 2-5 Technique of Direct Fist Percussion

nail. A rapid movement is necessary. (This will take practice!)

Direct and Indirect Fist Percussion

Refer to Figures 2-5 and 2-6. Note that the fist is either directly or indirectly applied to the organ and is used to assess tenderness. As mentioned previously, the reader

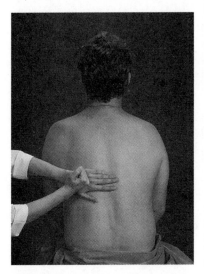

Figure 2-6 Technique of Indirect Fist Percussion

should know these techniques although they are rarely used with older persons.

Auscultation

To auscultate means to listen. Auscultation is accomplished either directly with your ear or indirectly with a stethoscope. Sometimes wheezes in a client with asthma are audible without a stethoscope. Most of the time a stethoscope is necessary (indirect auscultation) to distinguish abnormal from normal heart and lung sounds. Your stethoscope should be of average to excellent quality; as a result of improved technology, there are some very good devices that compensate for external interference sounds and focus on internal and clear soft sounds. The stethoscope has two major listening parts: the bell and the diaphragm. The bell is concave and used for low-pitched sounds; the diaphragm is flat and used frequently for all other sounds, including high-pitched sounds.

For the sake of the client's comfort, your own hands should warm parts of the stethoscope. A warm stethoscope connotes respect for the individual. The stethoscope does not need to be pressed snuggly against the skin, only comfortably placed; it will still pick up adequate sounds.

NURSING CHECKLIST

Physical Assessment Components

Inspection = look
Palpation = feel/touch
Percussion = tap and listen
Auscultation = listen
Intuit = sense/attend to

Figure 2-7 is a list of all the possible equipment used during a physical examination. The gerontological nurse may not use this equipment or have it available. You may need to rely on subjective data or the client's detailed stories and examples of clinical situations illustrating the health care status.

Equipment needed to perform a complete physical examination of the adult patient includes the following:

- Pen and paper
- Marking pen
- Tape measure
- Clean gloves
- Penlight or flashlight
- Scale (You may have to walk the patient to a central location if a scale cannot be brought to the patient's room.)
- Thermometer
- Sphygmomanometer
- Gooseneck lamp
- Tongue depressor
- Stethoscope
- Otoscope
- Nasal speculum
- Ophthalmoscope
- Transilluminator
- Visual acuity charts
- Tuning forks
- Reflex hammer
- Cotton balls
- Sterile needle
- Odors for cranial nerve assessment (e.g., coffee, lemon, flowers)
- Small objects for neurological assessment (e.g., paperclip, watch, pen)
- Water-soluble lubricant
- Various-sized vaginal speculums
- Cervical brush
- Cotton-tipped applicator
- Cervical spatula
- Slide and fixative
- Guaiac material
- Specimen cup
- Goniometer

The use of these items is discussed in the chapters describing the assessments for which they are used.

Figure 2-7 Equipment for physical examination

Summary

Inspection, palpation, percussion, and auscultation are the four components of physical assessment in the older adult. These methods are modified somewhat to accommodate the specific needs and conditions of older people. It is important to practice on colleagues to master the techniques described and to maintain sensitivity in how to adapt these techniques realistically to older people. Remember that the quality of life and wishes of the older person are first and foremost in any aspect of the nursing process.

References

Cauthorne-Burnette, T., & Estes, M. E. Z. (1998). *Clinical companion for health assessment and physical examination.* Albany: Delmar.

3

The Older Adult's Health History

Key Terms

advance directives
chief complaint
complete health history
elite older adult
episodic health history
genogram
review of systems (ROS)

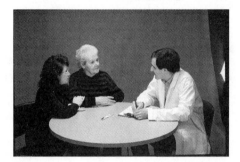

TIPS FROM THE EXPERTS

- If the older adult does not object, include family members/significant others if possible; they are valuable resources.
- Gain as much information and data as possible in advance.
- Kindness and patience with the older adult are well invested; they provide professional rapport and personal reward.
- Use conversational style to obtain data.
- Sit back and *observe* clients with dementia and cognitive losses; look beyond the words. Try to identify the *feelings* that they are conveying.

The health history on an older adult includes the rich complexities reflective of 60, 70, 80, 90, or more years of life experiences. Taking a health history on an older adult requires patience, caring behaviors, competency, communication, and coordination skills. The nurse must have the knowledge, awareness, and sensitivity to age-related changes that may affect the interview process to enable the older adult to share the rich history that has evolved over the years. Although there are four different classifications of health histories, the focus of this chapter is on the complete and episodic health histories, emphasizing the unique needs and concerns of the older adult.

tion on this chief complaint (**episodic health history**). On the other hand, the **complete health history** is a comprehensive compilation of data from a variety of sources in order to provide an in-depth profile on which to plan care. Circumstances requiring a complete health history include:

- Presurgical hospital admissions
- Nursing home admissions
- Home health care admissions
- Extensive long-term rehabilitative or chronic care

Refer to Table 3-1 for types of health histories.

Types of Health Histories

The process of history taking differs based on what necessitates the history. For example, if an older adult residing in a nursing home complains of indigestion, the nurse will focus questions and examina-

Sources and Issues about Data

Multiple sources are used in compiling the complete health history database on an older adult. *The most important source is the older adult.* Selective questions, progressing from general to specific, are

---

Table 3-1   Types and Characteristics of Health Histories

Complete health history
- Comprehensive
- Data on past and present health status
- Multidimensional
- Nonemergency
- Lengthy, in-depth

Episodic health history
- Based on a specific complaint or event
- Brief, specific data

Interval, or follow-up, health history
- Follow-up interview from an episodic visit
- Ensures recovery or treatment is altered to promote recovery or relief of symptoms

Emergency health history
- Basic, specific data obtained from multiple resources, often other than from the patient, in order to treat the emergency
- Minimal depth with focus on immediacy, quick resolution, or lifesaving treatment

---

Adapted from *Health Assessment & Physical Examination* (p. 40), by M. E. Z. Estes, 1998, Albany, NY: Delmar Publishers. Copyright 1998 by Delmar Publishers. Adapted with permission.

posed to the older adult. Even if the older adult is minimally able to respond, for example, because of aphasia or cognitive losses, it is vital that the nurse spends time interacting, observing, and establishing rapport. In addition, it is not uncommon for health care workers to *assume* that a physically frail or **elite older adult** (85 years and older) is cognitively not capable of verbalizing thoughts. In reality, it may be that the older adult is simply processing information more slowly and needs more time to respond, or, because of sensory losses, needs a modified approach. Modifications necessitated by age-related changes that older adults may need are listed in Table 3-2.

Because the older adult has collected a rich medical history over the years, it may be possible to access, by permission, a

Table 3-2   Unique Age-Related Changes as Expressed in Nursing Diagnoses and Nursing Interventions

Alteration in sensory-perceptual loss, risk for
- The nurse needs to ensure either hearing amplification or enhancement devices are in place and working.
- Distinctly articulate words; do not yell.
- Speak slowly (if you are a fast-paced nurse, this will be difficult).
- Speak in lower tones because with normal aging, the older ear hears lower tones more distinctly.
- Make direct eye contact.
- Sit at the same level as the older adult; do not tower over the older adult no matter what the position—in bed, in a chair, in a chair, or in a wheelchair.
- Use gentle touch to convey trust while recognizing that not every older adult is comfortable with touch.
- Clearly introduce yourself. First names convey warmth and informality in some cultures yet are inappropriate in other cultures.
- Smile; although this is a simple intervention, it conveys approval, comfort, confirmation, trust, security, and safety.

Activity intolerance, risk for
- Because the older adult may tire easily and have reduced energy levels, plan for rest periods.
- Two or more sessions may be warranted for the interview, along with one session for the physical exam and diagnostics.

Impaired mobility, risk for
- Allow for "stretch breaks" every 20 to 30 minutes; limb stiffness is normal.
- Do not use folding chairs; plan to use a firm, comfortable, yet supportive chair.
- Avoid chairs that are soft and low: they will be difficult to rise from.
- Keep walking devices, such as walkers, canes, and quad-canes, near by.

Impaired communication, risk for
- Arrange for the input/attendance of the older adult's significant other.
- Make paper and pencil available.
- Prior to the interview, consult with an occupational therapist and speech therapist for further suggestions on communication, if necessary.

continued

- If there is a language barrier and you are using an interpreter, review all questions with the interpreter in advance to assure accuracy.

Alteration in elimination patterns, risk for
- Allow for "bathroom breaks" every 30 to 60 minutes.

Fluid volume deficit, risk for
- Offer water as needed, but be aware of any fluid restrictions.
- Have high-liquid snacks available, such as gelatin and frozen ice pops.
- Avoid coffee and tea, which act as diuretics.

Alteration in pain, risk for
- Periodically ask the older adult if he or she is pain-free.
- Observe for signs and symptoms of pain, such as fidgeting, mild confusion, anxiety, or facial display indicative of distress.

Alteration in thought processes, risk for
- Politely redirect and return questions to health-related issues while affirming the value of the older adult's "story".
- Offer positive reinforcement (nodding "yes," valuing and confirming the feelings, empathizing, reflecting).
- Affirm life accomplishments that the older adult shares.

Impaired memory, short-term, risk for
- Give the older adult time to respond to questions pertaining to short-term events; although long-term memory remains intact, short-term memory diminishes.
- Give limited yet significant time listening to events from the past, with respect and interest.
- If the older adult expresses frustration about recalling events/data, reassure her or him to take time to recall or return to the question later.

Note: All are "risk for" diagnoses because these are normal or expected changes.

previous medical record. The record may provide "missing pieces" about lab work, immunizations, diagnostic testing, major and minor surgeries, a detailed history of falls, history of infections such as pneumonia or urinary tract infections, and medication history. Thus, the previous medical record may offer supportive data substantiating, refuting, or enhancing current findings. Note that the previous medical record is not a total replacement for the nurse's current findings; it may help to link and confirm other pieces of data. Remember, history tends to repeat itself; history of events and illness is important.

Significant others who reside with or who are familiar with the older adult are valuable sources of health-related data. They are able to observe the older adult on a day-to-day basis, making subtle observations in areas such as mobility and ambulation, prevailing affect (mood), and activities of daily living (ADLs). Interviewing these individuals separately, with the older adult's permission, encourages honesty and fuller data while preserving the dignity of the older adult. It also identifies emotional issues and needs of the significant other/caregiver who otherwise may not have the opportunity to reveal concerns and feelings.

Significant information is obtained from nurses, doctors, social workers, certified nursing assistants (CNAs), home health aides (HHAs), or other health care personnel who have previously cared for the older adult. For example, consider an older adult who, while living at home, managed his diabetes. Although he was able to correctly administer insulin, he was

NURSING TIP

Confidentiality of health-related data on an older adult or *any* client whom you are assessing has become more critical with the growth of technology. It is important to share client information only with pertinent members of the interdisciplinary health care team within a controlled environment. Computer printouts of the medical record should not be left unattended in the workstation. Computer passwords should be used for clinical reasons only and by designated personnel. In addition, as a variety of health care students, including nursing students, gain experience in the clinical area, guidelines on accessing client information "for learning purposes" must be established in order to maintain clients' rights and the confidentiality of these legal documents.

consistently nonadherent with dietary choices and preventive foot care—two significant health behaviors that affect the outcomes associated with diabetes. His home care nurse and home health aide are in ideal positions to provide data that identifies a learning need requiring further investigation. Circumstances and reasons for nonadherence would be explored during the health history interview.

On the other hand, consider another scenario: An older adult who has just been admitted to the nursing home was previously hospitalized for a total hip replacement. During the hospitalization, postsurgically on day 2, the older adult abruptly became confused, incoherent, and hostile, and physically fought with the nursing staff. Upon further investigation, the patient was found to have a toxic reaction from one of the medications. However, when the admission nursing staff queried the hospital nursing staff, the hospital staff recalled the patient to be "aggressive," to have "tendencies toward violent behavior," and to be "difficult to manage." This example illustrates that data can be inaccurate, biased, subjective, and situational as well as misleading if taken on face value.

Data from secondary sources must be treated suspiciously, scrutinized, and confirmed by examining the medical record and by questioning the older adult when obtaining the *current* health history.

Process of the Health History

The complete health history is conducted less frequently than the episodic health history, the latter of which is based on a **chief complaint.** The complete health history is a threefold process requiring planning, coordination, and therapeutic interview techniques:

- Demographic and background information is gathered in advance, if possible.
- The interview is arranged, in one or two hour-long sessions, depending on the energy level of the older adult.
- The **review of systems (ROS)** and physical examination are conducted separately; allow for approximately an hour together.
- If possible, a separate session is conducted sharing the results, concerns, implications for care, and recommendations of the nurse and health care team.

The total amount of time for a complete health history on an older adult may seem excessive. However, if the history is rushed, inaccurate false data will be obtained. Nursing care will then be based on inaccurate information, resulting in inappropriate care, ineffective, negative outcomes, and fictitious recommendations. This dangerous scenario holds the potential for harm and negligence, which could easily have been prevented by investing more time in the assessment phase, or foundation of care.

Interviewing the Older Adult

Therapeutic communication and facilitative interview techniques are tailored to the needs of the older adult. The result is a smooth flow of information and ultimate understanding of the health care needs of the older adult. Behaviors and symptoms associated with normal age-related changes as well as common diseases more prevalent in older adults must be considered during the interview process. The knowledge base necessary for understanding these changes and pathologies relative to the assessment of an older adult are covered throughout this book.

The interview environment (space in which the interview will occur) is selected and prepared in advance. Aim for privacy, comfort, and sufficient space with bathroom, beverage, and snacks at hand. Room temperature and ventilation should be adequate along with sufficient (at least 100 watt lighting, not 60 watt) lighting. Noise, distractions, and interruptions should be eliminated as much as possible. Interruptions or rushing the older adult devalues the older adult, minimizes effort, and promotes feelings of nonworth.

Optimum time of day for conducting a health history for most older adults is morning. Later in the afternoon or evening hours are not considered ideal times to perform cognitive assessments requiring memory, language, and recall tasks. Blood glucose normally fluctuates during these times, as do diurnal rhythms. In addition, many older adults manifest sleep pattern changes and retire for sleep earlier; they also wake up earlier. The elite (or frail) older adult may nap in the afternoon, because of lower energy levels. There are exceptions to these patterns based on the older adult's lifestyle. Individuals who were "night owls" at younger ages may continue with this pattern whereas "morning individuals" are likely to continue rising early. Ideally, ask the older adult which times work best for obtaining the health history.

When the older adult arrives for the interview, allow some time for acclimation to the interview environment. If sensory and cognitive losses are extensive, the older adult may become confused. The nurse should explain and reorient the individual. It is helpful to include the family or significant other as a means of support and familiarity for meeting the older adult's sense of security. If the older adult has a medical diagnosis of dementia, do not overwhelm him or her with excessive stimuli, detail, and conversation; observe, be there, and listen. The importance of just being there (your presence) is extremely important as a first step in establishing trust.

The nurse offers an introduction, including full name, and explains the purpose, sequence, and time frame of the interview. Conveying a professional image is part of the nurse's role. However, "professional" does not indicate "lifeless and solemn." In fact, emotional warmth and empathy are shown by means of body language and appropriate touch (a gentle handshake or touching the arm). Positive facial expressions and eye contact are also powerful communication interventions expressing support and security. However, be aware of cultural differences, which may convey the opposite meaning (Table 3-3).

The interview techniques summarized in Table 3-4 require the nurse's awareness and application. Initially, these techniques may feel uncomfortable and forced. As the nurse continues to use them, they will become more automatic.

Content of the Complete Health History

Tables 3-5 and 3-6 summarize the content of the health history. Again, the purpose is to obtain baseline data from which care will be planned. Although health history forms tend to be setting-specific, content remains the same. Certain sections, such as history of falls, functional and cognitive status, and medications, are examined more closely because of the far-reaching effects on the older adult. Modifications are made for the episodic health history that is driven by the chief complaint or presenting symptoms and conducted more frequently than the complete health history (explained and illustrated later in this chapter).

Table 3-3   Examples of Cultural Communication Differences

Asian Americans	• Tend not to express emotions • Use touch selectively • Do not verbalize extensively • Generally, are not confrontational • Use silence as a means of reflection • Are not receptive to immediate friendliness and display of caring feelings • Do not view eye contact as a positive gesture • Respect authority • Do not discuss intimacy and sexuality readily
Hispanic Americans	• Maintain eye contact comfortably • Respect endurance of pain • Value socializing prior to the task at hand, that is, the health history • Respond well to open-ended questions • Verbalize comfortably about intimacy and sexuality, if the nurse is the same gender • Detailed questions about family are not well received • Sense of time is carefree
Bulgarians and Tunisians	• Be aware that typical "yes" responses like nodding head vertically indicate "no" and "no" indicates "yes"
American Indians	• Interpret locked eye contact as negative • Use silence to reflect • Relate better if nurse is same gender when discussing sexuality • Do not readily discuss intimate matters • Are not comfortable with someone taking notes about what they are saying
African Americans	• Use moderate amounts of nonverbal gestures • Approach outsiders with caution • Are comfortable with eye contact • May question/challenge the nurse on issues being discussed

Adapted from *Health Assessment and Physical Examination*, (pp. 113–122), by M. E. Z. Estes, 1998, Albany, NY: Delmar Publishers. Copyright 1998 by Delmar Publishers. Adapted with permission.

Key Points on Demographics and Background Information

Demographic and background data provide a "sketch" of the older adult. It is useful if not essential to access the older adult's profile and background prior to the actual interview and physical exam. Obvious "red flags" or indicators are often revealed. Remember that these "red flags" are hypotheses or guesses until fully explored. Examples of indicators that may have health-related implications include:

Table 3-4   Communication Enhancers with Rationales, Related to the Interview with the Older Adult

Enhancer	Rationale for the enhancer
1. Greet the older adult using positive body language	Builds trust and rapport
2. Use appropriate touch	Shows warmth and caring
3. Introduce yourself: first name, last name, title	Demonstrates professionalism
4. Ask the older adult how she or he would like to be addressed during the interview	Values and respects the older adult's identity
5. Ask permission of the older adult for the presence of the significant other	Informs and promotes sense of security in the older adult
6. Explain the purpose, content, flow, and time frame of events of the health history	Same as above
7. Offer to meet the basic needs of fluids and toileting before you begin the interview	Prevents interruptions
8. Sit at an angle, side by side with the older adult	Holds attention
9. If hard of hearing (HOH), sit on the more functional side of the older adult	Individual has a better chance of hearing you without straining her or his neck
10. If eyesight is poor, maintain touch	The aging eye (presbyopia) has trouble accommodating to close objects due to lens inelasticity. Eye contact maintains rapport and attention.
11. Speak slowly, clearly, in low tones	The aging ear (presbycusis) has trouble discerning high-pitched sounds
12. Move from general to specific questions	General questions open up communication; specific questions capture needed data
13. Use open-ended questions to obtain in-depth data; close-ended questions for one-word, simple answers (yes-no)	Both in-depth and simple answers are warranted. "Tell me about your home" (open-ended question; it is general, and it opens communication). "Did you get a flu shot last year?" (close-ended; yes-no answer)
14. Apply therapeutic communication skills: attentive listening, clarification, reflection, restatement, silence	These techniques encourage more extensive responses with the intent of opening communication and thus gaining a fuller understanding of the history of the older adult.

continued

Enhancer	Rationale for the enhancer
15. Use "polite interruption"	Gently controls digressions; try not to use this technique when opening up communication
16. Periodically apprise the older adult of how much time remains	Encourages continued effort
17. Acknowledge the rich history being shared with you	Offers positive reinforcement; increases the older adult's sense of worth
18. Offer closure through summarizing briefly what was just accomplished through the entire health history	Reinforces the value of the older adult's life and time

- Date of birth (DOB): 1896
- Newly diagnosed with Parkinson's disease last month
- Started on levadopa two weeks ago
- Total number of medications: eight (polypharmacy)
- No living family
- History of wandering behavior times past six months
- History of three falls over the past month
- Has not determined **advance directives** (actions to be taken in the event of an incapacitating, disabling health episode) for care

Included in demographics is the category of occupation, previous or current. In many instances "retired" is listed as the answer. However, retirement is *not* an occupation. The term is nearly meaningless as a piece of data, and offers little substance; instead, seek data on the person's former occupation, and whether she or he continues to earn income from or volunteer in that role.

Medical diagnoses and list of current medications are often available in advance from the primary care provider or most recent health care encounter in the hospital, nursing home, or home health care agency. In addition, special dietary regimens and known allergies are obtainable yet need to be confirmed during the interview.

Family history, support networks, and ethnicity, including caregivers and community resource utilization, are critical in understanding the psychosocial and phys-

ical surroundings of the older adult. A **genogram** (Figure 3-1) may be accessed; if not construct one during the interview. The genogram is a visual blueprint, usually encompassing three generations, which includes disease history of one's parents, self and siblings, and one's children. The benefit of the genogram is that it is distinct and visible at a glance, insightful of genetic factors, and useful in estimating the degree to which family history has been influential in the older adult's health. In addition, prevention can be planned to offset some of the genetic factors. Remember that it may be impossible to obtain accurate and reliable data on the health care and diseases of the older adult's parents. Access to, type of, and quality of health care in the mid- to late 1800s was very different than it is currently. Similarly, data on childhood diseases and immunizations of the older adult may be vague at best.

Information on insurance coverage is usually accessible in advance and implies, to a degree, socioeconomic status. For example, if an older adult is on Medicaid, it can be assumed that economic resources and assets are limited. Also, most older adults are on a fixed income through Social Security, and are careful in budgeting monies for the month. Likewise, many have lived through the Great Depression of the 1930s when money was scarce, or other historical events such as confinement in concentration camps of Nazi Germany, which have deeply affected their lives. This background information is

Table 3-5   Content of the Complete Health History

I. Patient/client profile: age, sex, race, marital status, occupation
II. Reason for the health history interview
III. Present health and health practices. Frequency of:
   - Nurse Practitioner (NP)/primary care provider (PCP) visits
   - Eye, dental, hearing exams
   - Mammograms, GYN exams, pap tests
   - Breast self-exam
   - X rays and lab work: abnormal results
   - Current medications:
     - Generic and brand name of medications
     - Dosage
     - Frequency per day
     - Over-the-counter medications (OTCs) and usage
     - Whether the individual takes the medication at prescribed times or not (adherence, side effects)
     - Known hypersensitivity and allergic reactions to medications/foods/substances
     - Use and frequency of other substances: alcohol (ETOH), tobacco, illegal drugs (data from the client may be unreliable because of embarrassment or fear)
IV. Past health history:
   - Medical diagnoses
   - Surgical diagnoses (major)
   - Blood transfusions and blood type
   - Past medications: names of meds and reasons why not taking them
   - Communicable diseases: mumps, measles, childhood illnesses and immunizations
V. Family history
   - Construct a genogram
VI. Fall risk assessment and accident history
   - Assess safety judgment and awareness: ask, "What would you do if your apartment caught fire?" Examine degree of logic and safety judgment
   - Examine safety hazards (shower/bath hold bars, throw rugs, step stools, "rushing" behaviors)
VII. Functional status and assessment: ADL and instrumental activities of daily living (IADL) sample assessments in upcoming chapters
VIII. Mental status assessment: selective cognitive and affective assessment tools in upcoming chapters
IX. Sleep pattern assessment: subjective and objective data (quantity and quality of sleep)
X. Nutritional, hydration, and exercise status fluid intake and output (I&O) description of typical daily meals, likes and dislikes, dietary supplements and vitamins, activity levels, weight loss/gain within 5 pounds)
XI. Sexuality and intimacy assessment (perceived satisfaction with sexual expression, physical and emotional, "safe sex" practices)

continued

XII. Social history:
- Social support networks: internal (family and significant others) and external (community and home care resources)
- Travel, work, home environment, hobbies, leisure time activities
- Social skills
- Stress and coping skills (explore current and past coping methods)
- Education and literacy (ask person to read headlines and first few lines of a newspaper or large-print book)
- Socioeconomic status and issues
- Religious/spiritual practices: advance directives
- Roles and relationships (ask, "Tell me about those important persons in your life.")
- Self-perception ("How would you describe yourself?")
- Perception of overall health status ("Describe how you view your health.")

XIII. Review of systems (ROS) (12): Yes-no, close-ended questions according to body system, which indicates the presence or absence of a symptom or illness. Positive results are then used for further questioning (see Table 3-6).

Adapted from *Health Assessment and Physical Examination* (Chapter 3), by M. E. Z. Estes, 1998, Albany, NY: Delmar Publishers. Copyright 1998 by Delmar Publishers. Adapted with permission.

Note: Most nursing facilities, hospitals, and the like have their own computerized or preprinted forms.

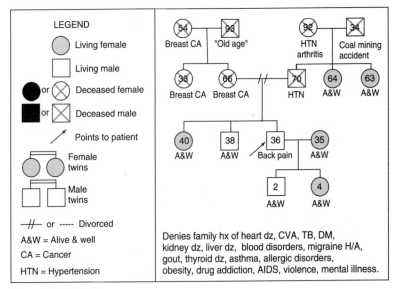

Figure 3-1 The Genogram

Table 3-6   Review of Systems

GENERAL
Patient's perception of general state of health at the present, difference from usual state, vitality and energy levels

NEUROLOGICAL
Headache, change in balance, incoordination, loss of movement, change in sensory perception/feeling in an extremity, change in speech, change in smell, fainting (syncope), loss of memory, tremors, involuntary movement, loss of consciousness, seizures, weakness, head injury

PSYCHOLOGICAL
Irritability, nervousness, tension, increased stress, difficulty concentrating, mood changes, suicidal thoughts, depression

SKIN
Rashes, itching, changes in skin pigmentation, black and blue marks (ecchymoses), change in color or size of mole, sores, lumps, change in skin texture, odors, excessive sweating, acne, loss of hair (alopecia), excessive growth of hair or growth of hair in unusual locations (hirsutism), change in nails, amount of time spent in the sun

EYES
Blurred vision, visual acuity, glasses, contacts, sensitivity to light (photophobia), excessive tearing, night blindness, double vision (diplopia), drainage, bloodshot eyes, pain, blind spots, flashing lights, halos around objects, glaucoma, cataracts

EARS
Hearing deficits, hearing aid, pain, discharge, lightheadedness (vertigo), ringing in the ears (tinnitus), earaches, infection

NOSE AND SINUSES
Frequent colds, discharge, itching, hay fever, postnasal drip, stuffiness, sinus pain, polyps, obstruction, nosebleed (epistaxis), change in sense of smell

MOUTH
Toothache, tooth abscess, dentures, bleeding/swollen gums, difficulty chewing, sore tongue, change in taste, lesions, change in salivation, bad breath

THROAT/NECK
Hoarseness, change in voice, frequent sore throats, difficulty swallowing, pain/stiffness, enlarged thyroid (goiter)

RESPIRATORY
Shortness of breath (dyspnea), shortness of breath on exertion, phlegm (sputum), cough, sneezing, wheezing, coughing up blood (hemoptysis), frequent upper respiratory tract infections, pneumonia, emphysema, asthma, tuberculosis

CARDIOVASCULAR
Shortness of breath that wakes you up in the night (paroxysmal nocturnal dyspnea), chest pain, heart murmur, palpitations, fainting (syncope), sleep on pillows to breathe better (orthopnea; state number of pillows used),

continued

swelling (edema), cold hands/feet, leg cramps, myocardial infarction, hypertension, valvular disease, pain in calf when walking (intermittent claudication), varicose veins, inflammation of a vein (thrombophlebitis), blood clot in leg (deep vein thrombosis), anemia

BREASTS
Pain, tenderness, discharge, lumps, change in size, dimpling

GASTROINTESTINAL
Change in appetite, nausea, vomiting, diarrhea, constipation, usual bowel habits, black tarry stools (melena), vomiting blood (hematemesis), change in stool color, excessive gas (flatulence), belching, regurgitation, heartburn, difficulty swallowing (dysphagia), abdominal pain, jaundice, hemorrhoids, hepatitis, peptic ulcers, gallstones

URINARY
Change in urine color, voiding habits, painful urination (dysuria), hesitancy, urgency, frequency, excessive urination at night (nocturia), increased urine volume (polyuria), dribbling, loss in force of stream, bedwetting, change in urine volume, incontinence, pain in lower abdomen (suprapubic pain), kidney stones, urinary tract infections

MUSCULOSKELETAL
Joint stiffness, muscle pain, back pain, limitation of movement, redness, swelling, weakness, bony deformity, broken bones, dislocations, sprains, gout, arthritis, osteoporosis, herniated disc

FEMALE REPRODUCTIVE
Vaginal discharge, change in libido, infertility, sterility, pain during intercourse, menses: last menstrual period (LMP), age period started (menarche), regularity, duration, amount of bleeding, premenstrual symptoms, intermenstrual bleeding, painful periods (dysmenorrhea), menopause: age of onset, duration, symptoms, bleeding, obstetrical: number of pregnancies, number of miscarriages/abortions, number of children, type of delivery, complications, type of birth control, estrogen therapy

MALE REPRODUCTIVE
Change in libido, infertility, sterility, impotence, pain during intercourse, age at onset of puberty, testicular pain, penile discharge, erections, emissions, hernias, enlarged prostate, type of birth control

NUTRITION
Present weight, usual weight, food intolerances, food likes/dislikes, where meals are eaten

ENDOCRINE
Bulging eyes, fatigue, weight change, heat/cold intolerances, excessive sweating, increased or no thirst, increased hunger, change in body hair distribution, swelling in the anterior neck, diabetes mellitus

LYMPH NODES
Enlargement, tenderness

HEMATOLOGICAL
Easy bruising/bleeding, anemia, sickle cell anemia, blood type

often passed on by the referral source (the person/provider who is referring the older adult for the complete health history).

Overall, demographic and background information accessed in advance provides skeletal data as a place to start in the quest for 100 percent accurate health-related data.

Modifications for the Episodic Health History

The episodic health history is almost the opposite of a complete health history. The complete health history is lengthy, multidimensional, and in-depth, whereas the episodic health history is specific and narrow in scope, seeking only pertinent information related to the chief complaint.

Consider the following scenario. You are caring for Mrs. Levy, and 80-year-old nursing home resident. Her medical diagnoses are congestive heart failure (CHF), peripheral vascular disease (PVD), hypertension (HTN) for 20 years, osteoporosis, and dementia, Alzheimer's type (late in the first stage). She ambulates effectively with a walker when she remembers to use it, otherwise she uses furniture for support. Her medications include Vasotec (enalapril), Colace, Maalox PRN, Milk of Magnesia PRN, Risperdal (risperidone), a multivitamin, and TUMS. At this point in time, Mrs. Levy is still a fairly reliable historian and is able to accurately verbalize discomfort and pain. She tells you, "My stomach is always bothering me. I always seem to have a stomachache. Can you help me, nurse?" Although you might be tempted to consider giving her Maalox PRN for stomach upset, *assessment must come first.* A brief episodic history should be included.

How should you proceed with Mrs. Levy?

- Warmly guide her to her room.
- Ask her if you can examine her stomach.
- Conduct an abdominal assessment (refer to Chapter 15).
- Pose some specific questions related

NURSING TIP

Never dismiss any individual's expression of discomfort or skip the step of assessing first. Even if there is data and reason to believe an individual's *memory* or *cognition* is impaired, it does not mean that *pain sensation* is impaired. In addition, another behavior associated with pain in older adults with later stages of dementia is increased confusion and rubbing or scratching at the site of pain.

to key aspects of the chief complaint, directed to location, radiation, quality, quantity, associated manifestations, aggravating factors, alleviating factors, setting, and time (Estes, 1998).

- Have you had this stomachache for a long time? (Ask her, even though this may be unreliable information: sense of time is one of the first aspects of orientation to change in dementia.)
- Describe the pain.
- Point to the pain and where it travels.
- Does the pain stay with you for a long time? Short time?
- Rate the intensity of the pain on a scale of 1–10—1 as least painful, 10 as maximum pain. (The older adult in this case probably will not be able to rate the pain; still try. Ask if the pain is "awful," "terrible," or "so-so" [average and bearable]. You must use terms/cliches that the patient can relate to.)
- Are you having other symptoms besides the abdominal pain? (Ask this question because stomach pain may relate to other body systems such as cardiopulmonary or genitourinary.)
- What gets rid of the pain?
- Does the pain ever stop? When does it stop? When does it start? Do you have it in the morning? At lunch? Supper? Breakfast?
- Does the pain make you double over at times? If yes, when?
- Review her medical record for gastrointestinal and cardiac-related clues.

The episodic assessment results in an intervention to treat or relieve the symptom. The nurse may have to collaborate with the physician or nurse practitioner for a diagnostic or pharmacological intervention. Even if the older adult has documented proof of relief from Maalox for the abdominal upset, it is absolutely paramount that the nurse makes a decision based on performing an assessment of related systems and a brief, episodic history.

Results of the Complete or Episodic Health History

The episodic health history ends with the nurse providing an intervention, then performing a follow-up interview to determine the outcome of the intervention. For example, if Mrs. Levy received Maalox for stomach discomfort, the nurse reexamines and questions the patient about degree of relief. However, with the complete health history, it is important to summarize conclusions and recommendations for comprehensive care planning. The family and older adult need to be present. Describe issues in simple, layperson's terms, which are understandable to the general public. In advocating for the older adult, the nurse needs to communicate on equal and practical terms.

Brief Introduction to the Physical Exam

The total physical exam is part of the complete health history and necessary to gain a comprehensive picture of the older adult's health. The nurse may need to schedule the exam after a break from the interview or on an entirely different day. The exam comprises **inspection, palpation, percussion,** and **auscultation techniques.** Detailed explanation of the physical examination will be covered in the following chapters as systems-related assessment is reviewed.

Thinking Critically about Health Data

For the most part, data is easy to collect; making sense of it is more challenging. Gaining a style of inquiry is a start in learning how to make connections related to care. Here are some suggestions on how to question and scrutinize data.

When thinking about health-related data, one should make connections and associations. It is associations that generate nursing diagnoses and eventual care planning. The triad of inquiry (Figure 3-2) is a simplistic method of prompting the nurse to think out loud. While examining any manifested clinical symptoms, the nurse concentrates on links in data between medical diagnoses/diseases and current lab work, asking how each is manifesting. For example, 89-year-old Mrs. Gomez has medical diagnoses of diabetes Type 2, osteoarthritis, and angina. Her medications are Precose (Acarbose) for the diabetes, Diuril (Chlorothiazide), and nitroglycerin s.l. prn. The inquiry process begins when the nurse asks herself the following questions:

- What are Mrs. Gomez's most recent blood glucose levels? What are the ranges? Does she get symptomatic when her blood sugar drops?
- How controlled is her angina? How frequently does she use nitroglycerin?
- Does she experience discomfort from the osteoarthritis? If yes, how does she relieve the pain?

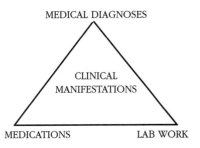
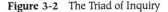

Figure 3-2   The Triad of Inquiry

- Why is she on Diuril? (She has no known diagnosis of hypertension. Moreover, hyperglycemia is a side effect of the thiazide group.)

Learn to *ask questions* of yourself and others, in order to link up data to care; do not be afraid.

Summary

The complete health history and episodic health history have been described and reviewed, including age-related differences and concerns. The nurse's application of sound interview techniques and effective accessing of data are the basis for facilitating the health history database. The nurse must examine sources of data with the suspicion of Sherlock Holmes, starting with hypotheses that need to be supported. For the episodic health history, the nurse focuses on the chief complaint and follows a line of inquiry toward the nine key aspects of the chief complaint. A summary of findings with recommendations for further investigation or care planning should always be presented to the family or client.

References

Estes, M. E. Z. (1998). *Health assessment & physical examination.* Albany: Delmar Publishers.

Taber's cyclopedic medical dictionary. (1997). Edition 18. Philadelphia: F. A. Davis Company.

4

Assessment of Vital Signs

Key Terms

apical pulse
blood pressure
brachial pulse
carotid pulse
dorsalis pedis pulse
femoral pulse
Korotkoff sounds
popliteal pulse
posterior tibial pulse
pulse
pulse deficit
radial pulse
rate
respiration
rhythm
temperature
temporal pulse
vital signs
volume

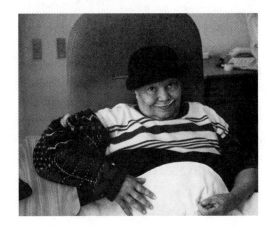

TIPS FROM THE EXPERTS

Accuracy of vital signs is essential. When teaching paraprofessionals to obtain vital signs, use demonstration and return demonstrations to ensure proper technique. Admission or illness-generated vital signs should be done by a nurse.

Don't rely 100 percent on numbers. Although number of respirations or blood pressure may fall "within normal limits," the client may still be in distress. Observe the client, look for symptoms of dizziness, confusion, discomfort, and overall well-being and factor this into your clinical judgment.

Traditionally, **vital signs** are known as "TPR and BP"—**temperature, pulse, respirations,** and **blood pressure.** Level of comfort/pain is considered a "fifth" vital sign and is critical as an all-encompassing signal of quality of life and well-being. Accurate findings and interpretation of findings provide information about the older person's baseline status. Equipment needed includes:

- Stethoscope
- Watch with second hand
- Thermometer (glass, electronic, tympanic; gloves and lubricant if rectal is the route)
- Sphygmomanometer
- Good hearing/vision (or compensatory devices) of the nurse

Physical and Psychological Presence

As emphasized previously, first impressions are important for understanding the client. Observation, conducted at eye level, includes paying attention to chronological age and apparent age. For example, many 90-year-olds look "young" for their age. Physically and psychologically they are coping and adjusting to age-related changes or chronic illnesses. They may have minimal wrinkles, healthy skin, well-cared-for teeth/dentures, and intact memory. In addition, they are active and ambulatory. In contrast, chronologically young adults—say, 66 years old—may present with wrinkled skin, sedentary lifestyle, and inactive mind and body. Systematically, the nurse observes for several parameters of "healthy aging":

- The nurse observes for hygiene and carriage. Is the older person well-groomed? If not, a mental notation is made to pursue a line of questioning surrounding this.
- What does posture look like? Does the person have kyphosis or scoliosis? Does the person carry herself or himself erect?
- What is the distribution of body fat? Is body fat equally distributed or located

on the midsection, upper arms, legs, or trunk?
- Is the gait smooth and steady? Or jerky and uncontrolled?
- Are there any body and/or breath odors? Food-related odors should be distinguished from hygiene or infection-related odors (very sour, very sweet, or very foul-smelling odors).

The above observations provide the hypotheses—the beginning guesses—about physical well-being of the older person. Psychological presence overlaps with physical presence; the two are integral or interconnected. Again, dressing, grooming, and hygiene are observed. Clean and neat is an accepted parameter of normality. Clothing should be congruent with climate, given cultural variations. Second, cooperation is a norm; if the client is uncooperative, find out circumstances surrounding this attitude. Third, question-answer responses to simple requests and simple small-talk conversation should be smooth and easy. If not, consider cultural and pathological possibilities. Remember that it is too early in the nurse's assessment to arrive at conclusions—just possible avenues of further investigation. Lastly, observe facial expressions—awake, alert, culturally appropriate, or not. These data provide further evidence for a variety of possible mental, sociological, and physiological issues as the assessment unfolds.

Comfort Level and Pain Perception

The degree of discomfort or pain can taint a first impression of a client. Besides this, for the client, pain influences quality of life. It is not necessary to live "in pain" and *no one* should have to. Therefore, it is paramount that the nurse determines the level of pain/comfort the individual perceives. Pain/comfort is subjective and must be assessed ultimately subjectively. (See Appendix H for pain assessment guidelines.)

Look for the following symptoms: labored breathing or speech; painful expression, given the person's cultural context; tearfulness, nervousness, or unwarranted laughter. In addition, observe for lack of eye contact, nail-biting, diaphoresis, or cold, clammy hands.

Sometimes, if the nurse simply "senses something is wrong," she or he should make a notation. There are times when a nurse cannot quite articulate or understand what is observed. These "feelings" should never be dismissed; what is seen or sensed in the client and the environment should be noted as a possible lead.

Temperature

Temperature is measurable body heat. Although rectal temperature is considered most accurate, it is also the most intrusive method of measurement. Oral, axillary, and tympanic methods are better ways of obtaining temperature.

Oral Method

The thermometer (glass or electronic) is placed under the tongue for 3 to 8 minutes or (electronic) until the beeping sound occurs. This method presumes that the client is able to adequately nose-breathe. Temperature is read and recorded. See Table 4-1.

Axillary Method

Axillary method requires placing the thermometer (glass or electronic) under the arm into the middle of the axilla. Keep in place 10 minutes. Use this time to talk with the client about health or psychosocial issues.

Tympanic Method

Cover the tip of the thermometer with the probe cover. Place over the ear canal. Tilt upward slightly, toward the opposite ear. Press start, then listen for the beeping sound. Remove from ear and read.

Rectal Method

Request that the older adult lie on her or his side with knees slightly flexed. Explain the procedure. Don gloves and apply water-soluble lubricant to the tip of the thermometer. Insert into the rectum approximately 1 inch/0.39 cm. Hold in place 3 to 5 minutes. Read and document.

Interpretation of Readings

Temperature is *not* a reliable indicator of infection in older people. A temperature of 100°C is alarming in an older person and may indicate serious infection or dehydration. Even temperatures of 99°F require examination of history of infection such as pneumonia and urinary tract infection (UTI). Altered body temperature may convey metabolic rate. For example, low resting temperatures may indicate hypothyroidism. Temperatures below 96.8°F (36°C) or above 100.4°F (38°C) should prompt concern and collaboration with the primary care physician or nurse practitioner to discuss etiology and interventions.

Pulses

Pulses, especially peripheral pulses, are difficult to find in some older people because of vascular disease. As the heart contracts, blood is ejected. This, in turn, creates movement of blood throughout the body. Heart rate, rhythm, and volume are noted.

Heart rate is number of heartbeats per minute. Sixty to 100 beats per minute are considered within acceptable limits. However, symptoms associated with the rates are most important. There are older people who feel "dizzy" with pulse rates of 60. In contrast, some complain of palpitations with pulse rates of 100. Always note subjective symptoms. Sites of palpating pulses are shown in Figure 4-1. Although nine sites are shown, two are used the most—radial and apical.

Radial pulse is found by palpating on the inner wrist, where the radial artery parallels the radial bone. Follow the thumb side of the inner wrist. Press the finger pads (first, second, and third fingers) against the radial artery with moderate pressure. If the pulse is irregular, count for a minute. If regular, count for 30 seconds and multiply by 2. It is not uncommon to discover irregular heart rates in older

Table 4-1   Advantages and Disadvantages of Four Routes for Body Temperature Measurement

Route	Normal Range	Advantages	Disadvantages
Oral Average 37.0° or 98.6°F	36.0°–38.0°C 96.8°–100.4°F	Convenient; accessible	**Safety:** Glass thermometers with mercury can be bitten and broken, causing client injury. Clients need to be alert and cooperative and cognitively capable of following instructions for safe use. **Physical abilities:** Clients need to be able to breathe through the nose, and be without oral pathology or recent oral surgery; route not applicable for comatose or confused individuals. **Accuracy:** Oxygen therapy by mask, as well as ingestion of hot or cold drinks immediately before oral temperature measurement, affects accuracy of the reading.
Rectal Average 0.7°C or 0.4°F higher than oral	36.7°C–38.7°C 100.8°F–104.0°F	Considered most accurate	**Safety:** Contraindicated following rectal surgery. Risk of stimulating valsalva maneuver in cardiac patients. **Physical Aspects:** Invasive and uncomfortable.
Axillary Average 0.6°C or 1°F lower than oral	35.4°C–37.4°C 95.8°F–99.4°F	Safe; noninvasive	**Accuracy:** Glass thermometer must be left in place for 5 minutes to obtain accurate measurement. Placement and position of thermometer tip affect reading.
Tympanic Calibrated to oral or rectal scales	See oral or rectal	Convenient; fast; safe; noninvasive. Does not require contact with any mucous membrane.	**Accuracy:** Research is inconclusive as to accuracy of readings and correlations with other body temperature measurements. Technique affects reading. Tympanic membrane is thought to reflect the core temperature.

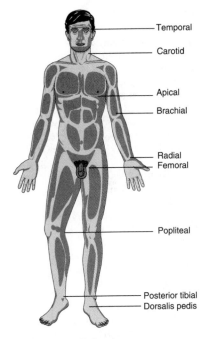

- Temporal
- Carotid
- Apical
- Brachial
- Radial
- Femoral
- Popliteal
- Posterior tibial
- Dorsalis pedis

Figure 4-1   Pulse sites

people. Irregular heart rates are *never* normal. Not all abnormal heart rates will be *treatable,* but must be identified for further investigation and discussion. Match radial with apical heart rate.

Use the diaphragm part of the stethoscope to auscultate **apical pulse.** The landmark is the left side of chest, left of the sternum, at the fifth intercostal space. Count the beats for 30 seconds, multiply by 2, for a regular rate; count 60 seconds for an irregular rate. When identifying the apex of the heart, note that in older adults, the heart may be slightly tilted left on its axis, placing it farther to the left. In addition, when identifying landmarks on older women, the nurse must move pendulous breasts. Do not use breasts as landmarks; use palpation of the ribs to find the fifth intercostal space.

The difference between the apical and radial rate is called **pulse deficit.** Apical greater than radial connotes a circulatory lag. In other words, there probably is a problem with circulation as the blood takes excessive time to get to the periph-

eral areas of the body. Listen to the apical rate separately, and then palpate the radial pulse. Subtract the difference.

Popliteal, posterior tibial, and **dorsalis pedis pulses** all evaluate lower extremity circulation, generally. These pulses may be difficult to palpate in older adults with circulatory problems or in those who have had surgery of the hips, knees, or legs. What is of most importance is to note when a pulse is absent. Doppler devices or other high-tech equipment may be used to determine presence of a weak pulse. At the same time as palpating the pulse, also feel for warmth, look for color of the extremity, and determine movement.

Rate, rhythm, and **volume** of pulses are usually noted. Rate is straightforward; it is number of beats per minute. Physiological changes, activity, emotional status, and environmental factors such as noise levels, pain, and mediations affect it. Rhythm is whether the pulse has equal intervals between each beat. The heart beats like the regular drumbeat of music. If "off-tempo" beats are found, they must be noted. These may be atrial or ventricular in nature, life-threatening or not, but must be further investigated.

Volume is not the beat but the pressure/amplitude exerted with each beat of the heart. Weak or bounding pulses are abnormal. Weak pulses may be due to shock or heart failure, whereas bounding pulses may be due to overexertion, fever, anemia, anxiety, hyperthyroidism, septic shock, or sometimes dehydration. See Table 4-2 for descriptors of pulse volume.

If in doubt about the "normalcy" of rate, rhythm, or volume of a pulse, weigh findings against what is considered normal—strong (not bounding), regular rhythm with rate between 60 and 100. Anything different than those findings begs for further investigation and collaboration with the health care team.

Respiration

A "respiration" equals one inhalation and one exhalation—breathing in oxygen and breathing out carbon dioxide. Respirations are counted and described. To count res-

Table 4-2   Scales for Measuring Pulse Volume

3-POINT SCALE

Scale	Description of Pulse
0	Absent
1+	Thready/weak
2+	Normal
3+	Bounding

4-POINT SCALE

Scale	Description of Pulse
0	Absent
1+	Thready/weak
2+	Normal
3+	Increased
4+	Bounding

pirations, discretely watch the rise and fall of the client's chest. One "rise and fall" equals one respiration. Similar to pulses, respirations are counted for a minute if irregular and 30 seconds multiplied by 2 if regular. Sixteen to 20 respirations are considered within the adult normal limits. Again, the nurse simultaneously must examine the whole individual—psychological distress, skin color, nature of the respiration (shallow or labored), diaphoresis, diaphragmatic retraction, and audible wheezing. (Chapter 8 presents a more thorough analysis of respiratory status in the older person.) From an experiential perspective, respiratory, cardiac, and abdominal episodic assessments are conducted *most* frequently given the common problems that older people exhibit. Chronic obstructive pulmonary disease (COPD), asthma, pneumonia, and cardiorespiratory-related illnesses such as congestive heart failure are common and challenge the respiratory assessment skills of the nurse.

Blood Pressure

Blood pressure is the pressure against the large arteries as blood passes through, somewhat like water through a garden hose. Systole and diastole are measured when taking a client's blood pressure (BP). Systole occurs when the heart contracts; diastole occurs when the heart relaxes. The arterial pressures during these two moments are represented by systolic and diastolic pressures, which are measured with a sphygmomanometer and relayed like a fraction (e.g., 120/70) in terms of millimeters of mercury (mm Hg). Blood pressure ranges for older people are the same as for younger adults. In general, hypertension should not go untreated in older adults. Hypertension is a dangerous yet treatable chronic disease; it is also a precursor to stroke. Therefore, it is essential that the nurse obtain an accurate pressure on the client. Classification of hypertension and blood pressure ranges are shown in Tables 4-3, 4-4 and Figure 4-2.

The more common site to measure blood pressure is the upper arm, where the brachial artery crosses the antecubital fossae. The thigh, above the popliteal artery, is another site of measurement but is rarely used. Sites to be avoided include:

- Painful limbs
- Arm at site of mastectomy
- Site of arteriovenous (AV) fistula or shunt (direct link between an artery and vein)
- Poorly perfused extremity
- Affected side from stroke

Size the individual's arm or leg for the correct size blood pressure cuff. Measure the circumference of the arm or leg to be used to take the blood pressure. Calculate two-thirds of the circumference. That number equals the size of the cuff, top to bottom (width of the cuff), to be used. Blood pressure readings in sitting, standing, and supine positions are taken to establish baseline data. Position the cuff as shown in Figure 4-3. Wrap the cuff completely around the upper arm with the bladder of the cuff deflated. Palpate the brachial artery and place the diaphragm of the stethoscope on the site. Pump the cuff to approximately 20 to 30mm/Hg above the previous reading. If a previous reading is unknown, pump the cuff to 160mm/Hg and listen for a sound. If no sound is heard, *slowly* release and listen for pro-

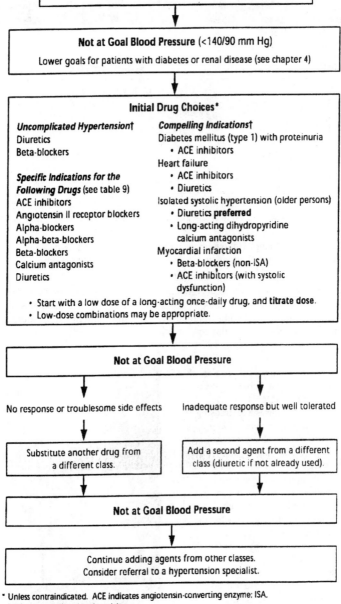

Begin or Continue Lifestyle Modifications

↓

Not at Goal Blood Pressure (<140/90 mm Hg)

Lower goals for patients with diabetes or renal disease (see chapter 4)

↓

Initial Drug Choices*

Uncomplicated Hypertension†
Diuretics
Beta-blockers

**Specific Indications for the
Following Drugs** (see table 9)
ACE inhibitors
Angiotensin II receptor blockers
Alpha-blockers
Alpha-beta-blockers
Beta-blockers
Calcium antagonists
Diuretics

Compelling Indications†
Diabetes mellitus (type 1) with proteinuria
• ACE inhibitors
Heart failure
• ACE inhibitors
• Diuretics
Isolated systolic hypertension (older persons)
• Diuretics **preferred**
• Long-acting dihydropyridine calcium antagonists
Myocardial infarction
• Beta-blockers (non-ISA)
• ACE inhibitors (with systolic dysfunction)

• Start with a low dose of a long-acting once-daily drug, and **titrate dose.**
• Low-dose combinations may be appropriate.

↓

Not at Goal Blood Pressure

↓   ↓

No response or troublesome side effects   Inadequate response but well tolerated

↓   ↓

Substitute another drug from a different class.   Add a second agent from a different class (diuretic if not already used).

↓

Not at Goal Blood Pressure

↓

Continue adding agents from other classes.
Consider referral to a hypertension specialist.

* Unless contraindicated. ACE indicates angiotensin-converting enzyme; ISA, intrinsic sympathomimetic activity.
† Based on randomized controlled trials

Figure 4-2 Algorithm for the treatment of hypertension (From *The Sixth Report of the Joint National Committee on Prevention, Detection, Evaluation, and Treatment of High Blood Pressure* [NIH Publication No. 98-4080], by the National Institute of Health–National Heart, Lung, and Blood Institute, 1997, Bethesda, MD: National Institute of Health.)

Table 4-3   Recommendations for Follow-up Based on Initial Blood Pressure Measurements for Adults

Initial Blood Pressure (mm Hg)*		Follow-up Recommended†
Systolic	Diastolic	
<130	<85	Recheck in 2 years
130–139	85–89	Recheck in 1 year‡
140–159	90–99	Confirm within 2 months‡
160–179	100–109	Evaluate or refer to source of care within 1 month
≥180	≥110	Evaluate or refer to source of care immediately or within 1 week depending on clinical situation

*If systolic and diastolic categories are different, follow recommendations for shorter time follow-up (e.g., 160/86 mm Hg should be evaluated or referred to source of care within a month).

†Modify the scheduling of follow-up according to reliable information about past blood pressure measurements, other cardiovascular risk factors, or target organ disease.

‡Provide advice about lifestyle modifications.

From *The Sixth Report of the Joint National Committee on Prevention, Detection, Evaluation, and Treatment of High Blood Pressure* (NIH Publication No. 98-4080), by the National Institute of Health–National Heart, Lung, and Blood Institute, 1997, Bethesda, MD: National Institute of Health.)

gression of sounds called **Korotkoff sounds** described in Table 4-5. Record BP as shown in the table.

If a Doppler ultrasonic transducer is used, gel for proper conduction is applied to the arterial site. The transducer is then placed over the site where Korotkoff sounds are identified. Immediately deflate the cuff completely after the process. It is not uncommon that while concentrating on the three BP numbers, the nurse may forget to deflate the cuff, creating discomfort for the client.

Blood pressure seems to vary with age. Nevertheless, high blood pressure should not go untreated because someone is "old." A blood pressure reading above 140/90 over three consecutive times warrants intervention.

The most common type of hypertension in older adults is systolic hypertension. Health teaching on cardiovascular health to reduce risk factors is paramount to controlling blood pressure. Smoking cessation,

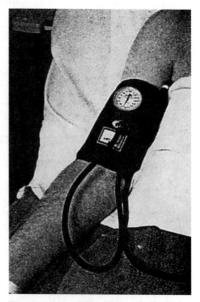

Figure 4-3 Appropriate Cuff Placement on the Arm

Table 4-4   Risk Stratification and Treatment*

Blood Pressure Stages (mm Hg)	Risk Group A (No Risk Factors No TOD/CCD)[†]	Risk Group B (At Least 1 Risk Factor, Not Including Diabetes; No TOD/CCD)	Risk Group C (TOD/CCD and/or Diabetes, With or Without Other Risk Factors)
High-normal (130–139/85–89)	Lifestyle modification	Lifestyle modification	Drug therapy[§]
Stage 1 (140–159/90–99)	Lifestyle modification (up to 12 months)	Lifestyle modification[‡] (up to 6 months)	Drug therapy
Stages 2 and 3 (≥160/≥100)	Drug therapy	Drug therapy	Drug therapy

For example, a patient with diabetes and a blood pressure of 142/94 mm Hg plus left ventricular hypertrophy should be classified as having stage 1 hypertension with target organ disease (left ventricular hypertrophy) and with another major risk factor (diabetes). This patient would be categorized as Stage 1, Risk Group C, and recommended for immediate initiation of pharmacologic treatment.

*Lifestyle modification should be adjunctive therapy for all patients recommended for pharmacologic therapy.

[†]TOD/CCD indicates target organ disease/clinical cardiovascular disease.

[‡]For patients with multiple risk factors, clinicians should consider drugs as initial therapy plus lifestyle modifications.

[§]For those with heart failure, renal insufficiency, or diabetes.

(From *The Sixth Report of the Joint National Committee on Prevention, Detection, Evaluation, and Treatment of High Blood Pressure* (NIH Publication No. 98-4080), by the National Institute of Health–National Heart, Lung, and Blood Institute, 1997, Bethesda, MD: National Institute of Health.)

weight reduction, stress management, and medication compliance are some of the dimensions of hypertension control. See Chapter 9, Cardiovascular Assessment.

Summary

Assessment of an older person's vital signs—TPR, BP, and comfort level—is a "compass" of the client's overall direction of health. Mastery of simple screening techniques provides baseline information for further in-depth appraisal.

References

National Institutes of Health, National Heart, Lung, and Blood Institute. (1997). *Sixth report of the Joint National Committee on detection, evaluation and treatment of high blood pressure*. No. 98-4080. Bethesda, MD: National Institute of Health.

For a copy of guidelines: http://www.nhlbi.nih.gov/nhlbi/nhlbi.htm

Table 4-5   Korotkoff Sounds

Phase I: This is the first sound heard upon slowly releasing cuff pressure. This sound represents systole and is recorded as the "top" number of the BP (e.g., 120/)

Phase II: Swishing sound heard as blood flows through vessels compressed by the cuff

Phase III: Beats become clearer and crisper in quality while still releasing cuff pressure

Phase IV: Beats become muffled; the first muffled sound is recorded as the first diastolic pressure reading (e.g. /80)

Phase V: Sounds cease; this is the second diastolic reading (e.g., 120/80/60)

Adapted from *Clinical companion for health assessment and physical examination*, by T. Cauthorne-Burnette and M. E. Z. Estes, 1998, Albany, NY: Delmar Publishers.

5

Skin, Hair, and Nails

Key Terms

acrochordon
actinic keratoses
arterial ulcers
cuticle
dermis
eccrine glands
ecchymosis
edema
elastosis
enterostomal therapy nurse (ETN)
epidermis
erythema
dermis
hirsutism
nail root
nailbed
periungual tissue
pressure ulcer
pruritis
ringworm
sebaceous glands
seborrhea
seborrheic keratosis
sebum
subcutaneous tissue
telangiectasia
turgor
Unna boot
venous ulcers
xerosis

TIPS FROM THE EXPERTS

A bronzed tan has been considered a sign of health and wealth. It is the role of the nurse to objectively inform older adults that "tan" is not equivalent to "healthy," and that there are hazards to overindulging in sunbathing. A sunblock at all times of *at least* 15 is recommended by dermatologists.

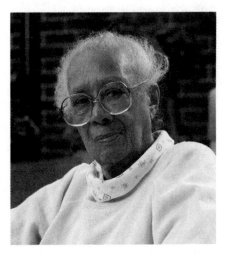

The saying "Beauty is only skin deep" rings true in Western society. Yet great importance and value are placed on the appearance of skin. In a youth-oriented society, smooth, wrinkle-free skin is considered beautiful, especially in women. Aspects of skin, hair, and nails related to health will be discussed in this chapter.

Basic Anatomy and Physiology

There are three layers of skin: **epidermis** (outer layer of melanocytes and keratinocytes), **dermis** (papillary and reticular layer), and **subcutaneous tissue** (connective tissue and fat cells). As people age, the subcutaneous tissue decreases and thins out. Skin thickness is between 0.2 to 1.5 mm, depending on the part of the body. In the elite older person, upon observation, skin appears paper-thin. Structures of the skin are shown in Figure 5-1. Refer to Figure 5-2 for structures of the nail.

Age-Related Changes in the Skin, Hair, and Nails

Refer to the accompanying box for age-related changes consistent with aging.

The dermatologist specializes in diagnosis and treatment of skin diseases. The plastic surgeon focuses on correction and reconstruction of the body, including the skin, bone, and soft tissues. Rashes and other skin abnormalities should not be ignored in older people; neither should the need for or desire of older people for reconstructive surgery. It is necessary that the nurse is aware of the health care team members for appropriate referral.

Inspection and Palpation of the Skin

In a well-lit room, observe for color, bleeding, cracking of skin, **ecchymosis**, vascularity, moisture, open areas, temperature, texture, **turgor** (tightness), and **edema**. Start from the head and work down.

Examine the face for rashes, raised areas, and consistency in color of eyelids,

AGE-RELATED SKIN, HAIR, AND NAIL CHANGES IN OLDER PEOPLE

Systemic changes: loss of cells, decreased circulation
- Loss of collagen (**elastosis**) and muscle, thinning, sagging skin, wrinkles
- Decrease in light-touch sensation
- Atrophy of subcutaneous tissue
- Hypertrophy of abdomen, thighs, and upper arms
- Decrease in sweat, **sebum,** and vitamin D production
- Diminished cell replacement
- Diminished response to skin injury

Loss of hair
- Hair thinning, graying
- Pubic, axillary hair thinning
- Decreased growth

Photoaging:
- Due to environmental damage; increases the appearance of "aging"
- Age spots
- Skin tags, benign (**acrochordons**)
- Fine wrinkling; leathery, lax, dry, blotchy skin
- **Telangiectasia** (dilation of small blood vessels, resulting in reddish vascular lesion)
- **Actinic keratoses** (skin tumor)— small scaly patches, pink to reddish
- **Seborrheic keratosis** (benign) epidermal growths

Dry skin: xerosis:
- Decreased moisture of the skin related to decreased **eccrine** (secretes sweat) and **sebaceous** (secretes oils or sebum) **glands**
- Itching (**pruritis**) and inflammation

Nails:
- Thicken, become brittle and hard
- Decrease in growth rate
- Develop longitudinal lines
- Dryness, uneven pigmentation

Adapted from Estes, M. (1998). *Health assessment & physical examination*. Albany: Delmar Publishers.

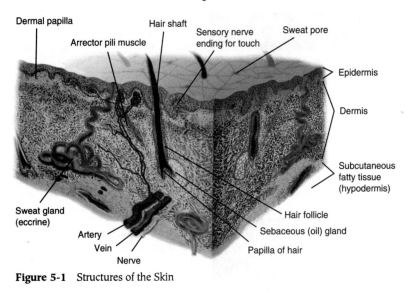

Figure 5-1   Structures of the Skin

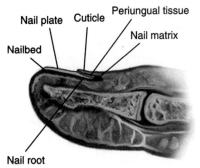

Figure 5-2   Structures of the Nail

Skin color indicating illness includes:

- Cyanosis (bluish) or ashen tint (in dark-skinned people)
- Jaundice (yellow, green, to orange hue, depending on underlying skin color)
- Hyperemia (bright red or pink coloration) consistent with infection, inflammation, or fever
- Polycythemia (bright red ruddy color) suggesting increased red blood cells
- Brown caste classically consistent with Addison's disease

nose, and ears. Lips and mucous membranes should appear shiny pink to deeper red or purple in persons of color. The neck, area behind the ears, arms, and dorsal and palmar surfaces of the hands should appear moist and free of discoloration and skin cracks. Apply gloves and examine torso, inguinal area, and genitalia, which should appear free from redness and swelling. Similarly, axillae, breasts, chest, legs, feet, and heels should appear symmetric and free from discoloration and open areas.

With the client positioned on the side, inspect the back, posterior neck, scalp, gluteal, and perianal areas.

Bleeding, ecchymosis, and vascularity are considered abnormal findings and should alert the nurse to clotting disorders, use of anti-thrombolytic agents, decreased platelet count, or increased venous pressure in superficial veins. When ecchymosis is discovered, abuse must be ruled out.

Increased familiarity with some commonly used descriptors of vascular skin findings is necessary in order to communicate those findings. Refer to the box on the next page

Lesions, if found, are identified by their anatomical location and whether they are localized, regionalized, or generalized. In addition, they are described as elevated,

⚠ NURSING ALERT

Signs of abuse in an older person may include black and blues or injury on the head, face, buttocks, breasts, abdomen, or limbs in the absence of a reasonable explanation. Burns and bite marks should also prompt immediate investigation. The client should be referred to the state ombudsman if *any* suspicion exists. State law varies.

TERMS COMMONLY USED TO DESCRIBE SKIN FINDINGS

Petechiae: specks (0.5 cm) of red-purple discoloration, nonblanchable
Purpura: hemorrhages into the skin; progresses from red, purple, and brownish-yellow; numerous causes
Venous stars: bluish vascular patterns, nonblanchable
Cherry angiomas: bright red areas, non-pathological
Port-wine stain: burgundy patch birthmark

Adapted from *Taber's medical dictionary*, 1995.

flat or raised, palpable or nonpalpable. Color, odor, measured size, and exudate (COME) should be noted. Identification and grouping of lesions are shown in Figures 5-3, 5-4, and 5-5. Skin lesions are considered an abnormal finding.

Palpation of the skin is always conducted using gloves. Skin is typically dry, yet if lesions, open areas, or drainage are present, gloves will protect the older person and the nurse from the infectious process. It is not uncommon to find dry skin (xerosis) cool to the touch in an older person, based on climate outdoors and in the home. Changes in the older person's body to adequately control temperature

result in cooler, warmer, and drier skin than that of a middle-aged adult. It is unusual to observe perspiration in many older adults as this mechanism is somewhat diminished, placing older persons at risk for heat exhaustion as well as hypothermia. Notably cool skin may also be caused by insufficient circulation, especially in the extremities. Disorders such as hypothyroidism must be ruled out as possible causes of cool, dry skin.

Testing for skin turgor is best accomplished by gently pinching and releasing the skin at the abdomen or anterior chest under the clavicle. Upon releasing the skin, it should quickly return to its original contour. Skin turgor in an older person is variable. In general, older individuals have less skin turgor than younger individuals because of the effects of gravity, decreased subcutaneous tissue, and sometimes disuse. Testing skin turgor helps to evaluate hydration status in a young or middle-aged adult, whereas skin turgor is not an effective measure of hydration/dehydration in an older person because of age-related changes in the skin and muscle.

Palpate for edema (fluid) in tissues by pressing your thumb against the skin and then releasing—especially in all extremities. Edema is described by the depth of the imprint:

- +0 = no pitting
- +1 = 0–1/4 inch pitting (mild)
- +2 = 1/4–1/2 inch pitting (moderate)
- +3 = 1/2–1 inch pitting (severe)
- +4 = greater than 1 inch pitting (severe)

Cardiovascular, renal, or lymph problems may interfere with fluid distribution and are possible causes of edema. Table 5-1 illustrates types of edema.

Some Skin Abnormalities

Skin cancers are common in older adults. Basal cell carcinoma, squamous cell carcinoma, and malignant melanomas comprise the majority of skin cancers. The box on page 48 describes characteristics of each.

LESIONS	EXAMPLES	LESIONS	EXAMPLES

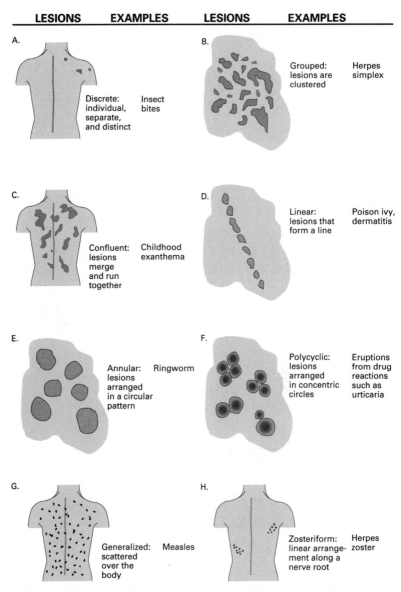

A.

Discrete: individual, separate, and distinct — Insect bites

B.

Grouped: lesions are clustered — Herpes simplex

C.

Confluent: lesions merge and run together — Childhood exanthema

D.

Linear: lesions that form a line — Poison ivy, dermatitis

E.

Annular: lesions arranged in a circular pattern — Ringworm

F.

Polycyclic: lesions arranged in concentric circles — Eruptions from drug reactions such as urticaria

G.

Generalized: scattered over the body — Measles

H.

Zosteriform: linear arrangement along a nerve root — Herpes zoster

Figure 5-3   Arrangement of Lesions

Wound Care Issues and Pressure Ulcers

Wound care is a fast-growing and expanding area of specialty relevant to assessment and care of older people. Delay in the healing of wounds in an older person is expected based on systemic changes in the immune system, nutritional status, functional status, and especially mobility. Generally, the better the overall health of the individual, the greater the

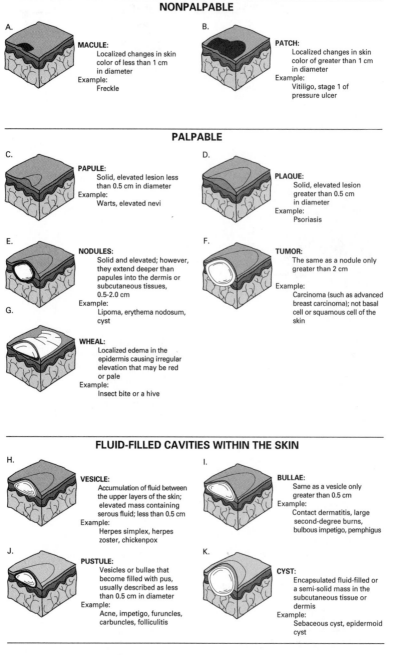

NONPALPABLE

A.

MACULE:
   Localized changes in skin
   color of less than 1 cm
   in diameter
Example:
   Freckle

B.

PATCH:
   Localized changes in skin
   color of greater than 1 cm
   in diameter
Example:
   Vitiligo, stage 1 of
   pressure ulcer

PALPABLE

C.

PAPULE:
   Solid, elevated lesion less
   than 0.5 cm in diameter
Example:
   Warts, elevated nevi

D.

PLAQUE:
   Solid, elevated lesion
   greater than 0.5 cm
   in diameter
Example:
   Psoriasis

E.

NODULES:
   Solid and elevated; however,
   they extend deeper than
   papules into the dermis or
   subcutaneous tissues,
   0.5-2.0 cm
Example:
   Lipoma, erythema nodosum,
   cyst

F.

TUMOR:
   The same as a nodule only
   greater than 2 cm

Example:
   Carcinoma (such as advanced
   breast carcinoma); not basal
   cell or squamous cell of the
   skin

G.

WHEAL:
   Localized edema in the
   epidermis causing irregular
   elevation that may be red
   or pale
Example:
   Insect bite or a hive

FLUID-FILLED CAVITIES WITHIN THE SKIN

H.

VESICLE:
   Accumulation of fluid between
   the upper layers of the skin;
   elevated mass containing
   serous fluid; less than 0.5 cm
Example:
   Herpes simplex, herpes
   zoster, chickenpox

I.

BULLAE:
   Same as a vesicle only
   greater than 0.5 cm
Example:
   Contact dermatitis, large
   second-degree burns,
   bulbous impetigo, pemphigus

J.

PUSTULE:
   Vesicles or bullae that
   become filled with pus,
   usually described as less
   than 0.5 cm in diameter
Example:
   Acne, impetigo, furuncles,
   carbuncles, folliculitis

K.

CYST:
   Encapsulated fluid-filled or
   a semi-solid mass in the
   subcutaneous tissue or
   dermis
Example:
   Sebaceous cyst, epidermoid
   cyst

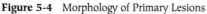

Figure 5-4   Morphology of Primary Lesions

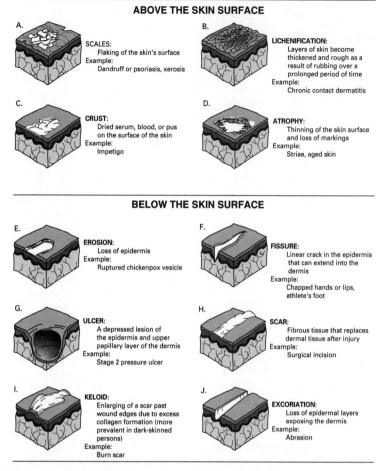

ABOVE THE SKIN SURFACE

A.
SCALES:
Flaking of the skin's surface
Example:
Dandruff or psoriasis, xerosis

B.
LICHENIFICATION:
Layers of skin become thickened and rough as a result of rubbing over a prolonged period of time
Example:
Chronic contact dermatitis

C.
CRUST:
Dried serum, blood, or pus on the surface of the skin
Example:
Impetigo

D.
ATROPHY:
Thinning of the skin surface and loss of markings
Example:
Striae, aged skin

BELOW THE SKIN SURFACE

E.
EROSION:
Loss of epidermis
Example:
Ruptured chickenpox vesicle

F.
FISSURE:
Linear crack in the epidermis that can extend into the dermis
Example:
Chapped hands or lips, athlete's foot

G.
ULCER:
A depressed lesion of the epidermis and upper papillary layer of the dermis
Example:
Stage 2 pressure ulcer

H.
SCAR:
Fibrous tissue that replaces dermal tissue after injury
Example:
Surgical incision

I.
KELOID:
Enlarging of a scar past wound edges due to excess collagen formation (more prevalent in dark-skinned persons)
Example:
Burn scar

J.
EXCORIATION:
Loss of epidermal layers exposing the dermis
Example:
Abrasion

Figure 5-5 Morphology of Secondary Lesions

likelihood of faster wound healing. Wounds influence an individual's body image and therefore sensitivity to the psychosocial aspects of having a wound is important to wholistic interventions.

A wound is a break or injury in the skin or soft parts of body tissue caused by any of the following:

- Trauma
- Surgery
- Pressure, shearing, friction, or moisture
- Puncture
- Laceration
- Perforation, crushing
- Severe inflammation or severe edema

Chronic wounds and pressure ulcers are the most common wounds in older adults. Steps in the assessment of wounds, pressure ulcers, and venous versus arterial ulcers are listed in the box on page 49, and Tables 5-2 and 5-3. The Braden scale for predicting risk is found in the Appendix.

SKIN CANCERS IN OLDER PEOPLE

Basal cell carcinoma
- Slow-growing
- Metastases are rare
- Associated with sun exposure
- Raised and waxy in appearance
- Nose, eyelid, cheek, or trunk are common sites
- Microsurgery for removal

Squamous cell carcinoma
- Slow-growing
- Scaly, elevated lesion
- Irregular shape; may bleed
- May metastasize
- Microsurgery for removal

Malignant melanoma
- Develops from melanocytes
- Change in mole or bleeding may occur
- Back and lower extremities are common sites
- May metastasize
- Deep surgical removal, chemotherapy, and/or radiation therapy
- Follow-up exams are essential

Adapted from Estes, M. (1998). *Health assessment & physical examination.* Albany: Delmar Publishers.

Inspection and Palpation of the Hair

Color of hair and presence and distribution of lesions of the scalp are noted during inspection and palpation of hair and scalp. Melanin decreases with aging and therefore gray hair is generally found throughout the body of an older client. Eyelashes, eyebrows, and scalp hair will be gray unless chemically treated. Thinning of scalp, axillary, and pubic hair is a common finding. Hair is evenly and bilaterally distributed. Factors such as presence of endocrine disorders, autoimmune diseases, severe stress, infection, chemotherapy, or radiation therapy tend to decrease hair growth and alter distribution. Hair texture may vary. Brittle hair may indicate malnutrition or chemical treatment. **Hirsutism** (excessive hair) may be present, caused by increased adrenal function due to pathology or medications.

Observe for **ringworm** (dermatomycosis), especially of the scalp (tinea capitis), lesions, or dandruff (**seborrhea**). Ringworm presents as a ringed patch, reddish and with vesicles and scaling. It is accompanied by itching and some pain. Head lice (pediculosis capitis) appear like dandruff, only the white flecks are attached to

Table 5-1   Types of Edema

Type	Location
Pitting	Edema that is present when an indentation remains on the skin after applying pressure
Nonpitting	Edema that is firm with discoloration or thickening of the skin; results when serum proteins coagulate in tissue spaces
Angioedema	Recurring episodes of noninflammatory swelling of skin, brain, viscera, and mucous membranes; onset may be rapid with resolution requiring hours to days
Dependent	Localized increase of extracellular fluid volume in a depenent limb or area
Inflammatory	Swelling due to an extracellular fluid effusion into the tissue surrounding an area of inflammation
Noninflammatory	Swelling or effusion due to mechanical or other causes not related to congestion or inflammation

ASSESSMENT OF WOUNDS

Size

- Diameter, circumference, or trace of the wound
- Depth

Surrounding Skin

- Moisture
- Color
- Suppleness

Wound bed; identify:

- Granulation tissue
- Necrotic tissue
- Fibrin, slough
- Epithelium
- Exudate
- Odor

Wound edges

- Inspect outline of the edges
- Undermining

Adapted from Krasner, D. & Kane, D. (1997). *Chronic wound care: A clinical source book for healthcare professionals* (2nd ed.). Wayne, PA: Health Management Publications, Inc.

the hair shaft and are not easily removed. Similarly, scabies (the "itch mite") infests areas such as between fingers, between toes, axillae, thighs, and genitals. The skin

⍰ NURSING ALERT

Do not use donut-cushion devices; they constrict blood flow.
Do not massage bony prominences; this damages tissues.
Do not overuse soap; this dries skin.
Provide good hygiene for incontinent clients *at the time of soiling.*
Generally, avoid the use of alcohol, peroxide, or betadine as a skin treatment.
Assess skin *daily.*
Ambulate. Provide passive or active range of motion.

⍰ NURSING ALERT

Many older people should not attempt to clip their toenails. Those with chronic systemic diseases such as diabetes or with leg ulcers or peripheral vascular disease should make regular visits (every 3 to 6 months) to the podiatrist. The gerontological nurse's awareness and application of skin, foot, and nail care can prevent loss of an older adult's limb.

appears to have numerous pustules and vesicles resulting in eczema. Repeated topical treatments clear these skin infections.

These skin infections have negative connotations for many older adults, indicative of poor hygiene and an unclean environment, which is not necessarily the case. Ringworm, for example, is carried by fungi and a parasitic insect carries head lice transmitted through common use of infected brushes and combs.

It is paramount that issues of body image and self-esteem are addressed, as they relate to what is considered normative and acceptable to the older individual and society. Moreover, many skin problems are not only curable but also cosmetically correctable. Just because people are older does not mean that they value their appearance less.

Inspection and Palpation of the Nails

Color, shape, configuration, and texture are assessed. Determine that the nails are not extensions or "fake"; also, any nail polish should be removed for accurate assessment. If possible, arrange to reapply the polish after the assessment as a courtesy to the individual.

Fingernails and toenails are inspected for capillary refill, leukonychia (white discoloration suggesting trauma, infection, anemia, or hypercalcemia), splinter hemorrhages (suggests endocarditis; mitral stenosis), or clubbing (suggests hypoxia). Refer to Figures 5-7 and 5-8.

Table 5-2   Stages of Pressure Ulcers and Treatment (AHCPR guidelines)

Stage	Treatment
Stage I : • Redness (**erythema**) of skin • Nonblanchable • Usually over bony prominences • Warm, swelling, discoloration, and hardness of area, in dark-skinned people	• Relieve pressure (pressure-reducing mattresses, wedge cushioning) • Turn frequently (every 2 hours at least) • Reduce friction, shear, moisture • Adequate food, calories, and fluid, especially protein, zinc, vitamin C, and water
Stage II: • Epidermis and dermis is involved • Blister-like • Superficial tear	TX: • Hydrocolloid dressing
Stage III: • Subcutaneous tissue to fascia involved • Possibly undermining of surrounding tissue	TX: • Prevent/treat infection • Debridement, mechanically or enzymatically, if necessary • Products to keep wound bed moist
Stage IV: • Damage to muscle and bone or tendons • Undermining and possible sinus tracts	TX: • Surgical reconstruction, debridement • Prevention of osteomyelitis • Products to keep the wound bed moist

Note: If necrotic tissue is present, it must be debrided before staging.

Palpate the nails with thumb and index finger for degree of firmness. The nail should not be spongy or easily bendable. Cardiac and respiratory diseases such as chronic bronchitis and emphysema contribute to weak nails.

Health Teaching and Prevention

Skin problems are preventable through the gerontological nurse's commitment to client, caregiver, and group education (i.e., senior and assisted living centers). Area dermatologists, **enterostomal therapy nurses (ETN),** and podiatrists are of-

ten willing to join in the campaign for skin cancer prevention. Collaborative efforts tend to reach more people than singular efforts.

The consequences of Lyme disease may include facial paralysis, palpitations, and debilitating joint inflammation. Treatment includes a 3-week course of antibiotics. Prevention comprises a three-shot vaccine, use of tick repellent, and light-colored long-sleeve and long-pant clothing with tight cuffs and pant legs. Inspection for ticks should occur after going outdoors. If found, remove the tick by its head, place it in a plastic bag, and show it to the physician or nurse practitioner.

Table 5-3 Quick Comparison of venous versus arterial ulcers	
Venous ulcers	**Arterial ulcers**
Cause: venous insufficiency Location: middle of the leg, large ulcers, edematous, less painful than arterial ulcers	Cause: ateroslerosis Location: lateral aspect of the leg or ankles, painful, appearing purple, patchy, cold, clammy, toenails distorted and thick, absence or weak pulses • Shiny and smaller than venous ulcers, clearly demarcated
TX: • compression stocking, elevate feet, vitamin C, zinc, control and management of disease • polyurethane foam dressing, steroid ointment or occlusive dressing, **Unna boot** (pressure wrap, applied about once weekly). • If cellulitis, antibiotics are used	TX: • Reduce/stop smoking, and foods that cause vasoconstriction • Control hypertension and obesity • Refer to podiatrist

Health care providers should not assume that older adults are not susceptible to this disease because of inactivity or place of residence. Day-trips as well as visiting family or gardening place them at risk. Good skin assessment and client teaching can promote early detection and treatment. For more information, visit the National Institute of Allergy and Infectious Disease website.

Teaching skin self-assessment to an older person and family member is a valuable and lifesaving skill. The accompanying boxes provide you with teaching guidelines. Visit the American Cancer Society website for further information.

Summary

Examination of the skin of the older adult will uncover treatable and, in many instances, curable problems. Age-related changes in the skin can be significantly yet partially controlled through awareness and client education. Limiting sun exposure and wearing proper clothing are two critical strategies to reduce the risk of skin cancer. Especially in the nursing home population, pressure ulcer assessment and staging are essential to prevention and appropriate treatment.

> ### ⚉ NURSING ALERT
>
> Lyme disease, one of several tick-borne diseases, can become debilitating. It is most prevalent in the Northeast United States. The symptoms include:
>
> • Circular rash with small white lumps
> • Flu-like symptoms
> • Swollen glands and joints

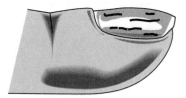

Figure 5-7   Splinter Hemorrhages

Normal nail angle

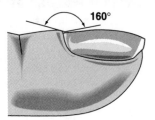

160°

Curved nail
variant
of normal

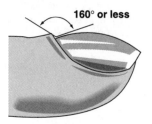

160° or less

Early clubbing

180°

Figure 5-8   Nail Angles

References

Krasner, D., & Kane, D., editors (1997). *Chronic wound care: A clinical source book for healthcare professionals* (2nd ed.). Wayne, PA: Health Management Publications, Inc.

SKIN CANCER PREVENTION GUIDELINES

Ultraviolet radiation from the sun is responsible for the majority of skin cancers.

1. Wear a sunblock of at least 15 when outdoors, even on cloudy or hazy days. Apply at least 45 minutes before going outdoors and reapply as directed. Do not forget to apply sunblock to feet if wearing sandals, and to ears, if exposed. Wear sunglasses to protect the eyes.
2. Avoid midday sun.
3. Avoid tanning and tanning booths.
4. Wear brimmed light-colored hats and protective clothing.
5. At your annual physical examination, remind your physician or nurse practitioner to inspect any suspicious moles.
6. Adequate vitamins (A, D, E) and water (eight to ten 8 ounce glasses daily) promote healthy skin.

Panel for the Prediction and Prevention of Pressure Ulcers in Adults. (1992). *Pressure Ulcers in Adults: Prediction and Prevention. Clinical Practice Guideline, Number 3.* AHCPR Publication No. 92-0047. Rockville, MD: Agency for Health Care Policy and Research, Public Health Service, U.S. Dept. of Health and Human Services. May 1992. [most recent as of May 2000] *For copies call 1-800-358-9295.

Sussman, C. (1999). *Wound care: Patient education resource manual.* Gaithersburg: Aspen Publishers.

Zator Estes, M. (1998). *Health assessment & physical examination.* Albany: Delmar Publishers.

SKIN SELF-ASSESSMENT

Observe for abnormally shaped moles, large (greater than the diameter of a pencil eraser) moles, bleeding moles, and moles of a color other than brown or dark brown.

1. Instruct the client to ensure that the room is well-lit.
2. A hand-held mirror and full-length mirror are necessary equipment if the older person does not have a significant other.
3. Outstretch the hands and arms, palm up, and inspect from fingers to forearms.
4. Inspect the backs of the hands and arms by bending both arms up and facing the mirror.
5. Unclothed, stand in front of a full-length mirror and inspect your body top to bottom, several times. Face to the left and right sides, raise arms and inspect, top to bottom several times.
6. Stand with your back to the mirror and using a hand-held mirror inspect the upper back, waist to back of the neck.
7. Observe the back of legs and buttocks, by standing with your back to the mirror, peering backward.
8. With one hand, part small portions of the hair. Use the other hand to position the hand-held mirror to inspect the scalp. View the back of the head by repeating this procedure, only this time with your back facing the full-length mirror.
9. While sitting down, use the hand-held mirror to examine the inner legs and heels.

Note: Many of these positions may be difficult to achieve and therefore recruit a friend or significant other with whom you are comfortable.

Adapted from Sussman, C. (1999). *Wound care: Patient education resource manual.*

6

Head and Neck Assessment

Key Terms

acromegaly
Bell's Palsy
bruits
cachexia
Graves' Disease
extrapyramidal
frontal area
goiter
hyperthyroidism
hypothyroidism
iatrogenic
lipoma
myxedema
occipital area
osteomyelitis
parietal area
self-care deficit
sternocleidomastoid muscles
tardive dyskinesia
temporal area
temporomandibular joint
torticollis

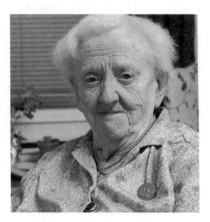

TIPS FROM THE EXPERTS

Lack of cleanliness of the hair and scalp may indicate a **self-care deficit.** Limited range of motion in the arms, reduced dexterity in fingers and hands, and reduced movement in the neck contribute to difficulty in shampooing and brushing the hair and scalp. Ask the older adult to describe such care, then intervene to improve self-care ability. Self-care includes activities of daily living such as eating, dressing, grooming, bathing and toileting.

Assessment of the head and neck of an older adult can reveal many different medical problems. Inspection and palpation are the main methods of examination employed, resulting in objective data contributing to the assessment database. In addition, the older adult is interviewed to obtain subjective data related to problems of the head and neck, such as history of headaches, sinus infection, thyroid dysfunction, or arthritis.

Figures 6-1, 6-2, and 6-3 depict bones of the face and skull, thyroid gland area, and lymph nodes of the head and neck, respectively. Familiarity with these landmarks is paramount to physical examination and assessment.

When inspecting or palpating the head and neck, it is essential to consider the mental status of the older adult. For example, if the older adult is fearful, or paranoid, or has a history of abuse or dementia, she or he may respond in an unpredictable manner. It is helpful to elicit the support of a family member in creating a safe and secure environment.

Inspection

Symmetry of the head is a normal finding. As the nurse faces the older adult, protrusions, bulges, swelling, or enlargements signal injury or presence of a mass. A summary of normal findings is listed in Table 6-1.

Enlargement of features (**acromegaly**)

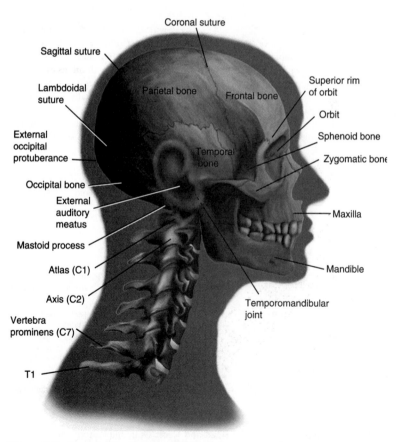

Figure 6-1   Bones of the Face and Skull

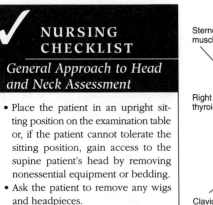

NURSING CHECKLIST

General Approach to Head and Neck Assessment

- Place the patient in an upright sitting position on the examination table or, if the patient cannot tolerate the sitting position, gain access to the supine patient's head by removing nonessential equipment or bedding.
- Ask the patient to remove any wigs and headpieces.
- Always compare the right and left sides of the head, neck, and face.

is an abnormal finding and is related to increased pituitary function and release of growth hormone.

Bell's Palsy, a condition of facial nerve damage, is another abnormal finding that may be mistaken for a cerebral vascular accident. See Figure 6.4.

Facial expression connotes level of physical and mental health, including subtle manifestations of medication or substance misuse. Look for a flat affect, frown-

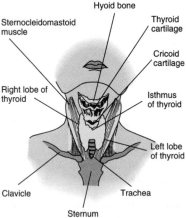

Figure 6-2 Thyroid Gland and Surrounding structures

ing, downcast eyes, or facial tension, all of which warrant further investigating of their causes. Be mindful that psychotropic and anti-Parkinson medications may affect facial expressions. Assessment of cranial nerves V and VII are usually conducted at this time. See Chapter 12.

Involuntary facial or head movement is an abnormal finding and may indicate **ex-**

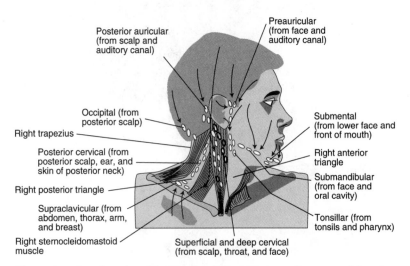

Figure 6-3 Lymph nodes of the Head and Neck: Drainage Patterns and Anterior and Posterior Cervical Triangles

Table 6-1   Normal Age-Related Findings Related to Head and Neck Examination

- Shortening in neck due to vertebral wear and tear
- Atrophy of face and neck muscles
- Presence of a "buffalo hump" at top of cervical vertebrae
- Reduced range of motion of head and neck
- Decrease in salivary gland secretion
- Thinning and graying of hair

Adapted from Burke, M., & Walsh, M. (1997). *Gerontologic nursing: Wholistic care of the older adult.* St Louis: Mosby.

trapyramidal activity or **tardive dyskinesia,** an **iatrogenic** disease associated with psychotropic drug usage.

Presence of facial edema may indicate sodium and/or fluid retention. Causes may range from ingestion of a high-sodium diet to cardiac or kidney disease.

Endocrine problems, such as **myxedema** (associated with **hypothyroidism** and **Graves' Disease, hyperthyroidism,** and increases in T_3 and T_4 blood levels), are discovered upon inspection by an astute clinician. In addition,

cachexia and **torticollis** may be noted. Cachexia is a wasting or emaciation of the body. Torticollis is a lateral deviation of the neck due to a congenital abnormality, hematoma, muscle spasm, or cholinergic activity. Both are noted in Figures 6-5 and 6-6.

Palpation

Use the pads of the fingers to gently palpate the scalp for lumps. Begin with both hands at the **frontal** area proceeding to **parietal, temporal,** and **occipital** sections of the head. The skull is smooth; masses of any type usually constitute an abnormal finding. Also, if the skull feels unusually soft upon palpation, **osteomyelitis** might be suspected due to extension of an untreated sinus infection. Pain upon palpation should be noted and further investigated.

Inspect the scalp by repeatedly separating the hair. Hair thinning and graying is part of normal aging. The scalp should appear clean, residue-free, and shiny. Sebaceous cysts may be noted; although benign, they do warrant notation and further investigation by a dermatologist.

Bilaterally palpate the **temporomandibular joint** located anteriorly to the tragus of the ear as the older adult opens and closes his or her mouth. Note any discomfort, clicking, or crepitus.

As the focus of the exam shifts to the

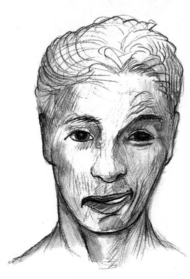

Figure 6-4   Bell's Palsy

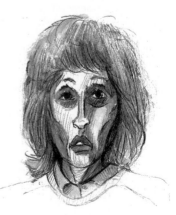

Figure 6-5   Cachectic Face

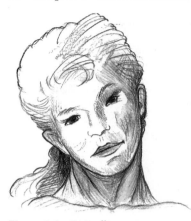

Figure 6-6   Torticollis

neck, symmetry of the musculature con-
stitutes normal findings. **Sternocleidomastoid muscles** and trapezii should appear symmetrical. Upon palpation, there
should be no masses or discomfort. Ask
the older adult to move the head side to
side as well as back and forward, and to
touch chin to chest. It is not uncommon to
find moderate to severe limitations in
movement due to osteoporosis, kyphosis,
scoliosis, arthritis, degenerative joint disease, or history of neck injury.

Assessment of the thyroid requires facing and inspecting the older adult as sips
of water are swallowed. No noticeable
movement should be noted in the front of
the neck. In males, thyroid cartilage movement may be prominent (movement of
Adam's apple). **Goiter**, an enlarged thyroid, is an indication of thyroid disease,
warranting diagnostic testing.

Palpation of the thyroid is conducted
posteriorly. The nurse stands behind the
seated client and with thumbs on the back
of the client's neck, places his or her fingers anteriorly on the section over the
lower trachea. Ask the client to take sips
of water. Assess for nodules and tenderness in conjunction with movement of the
gland. Palpate each side separately by se-
curing the trachea with finger pads of one
hand while palpating the thyroid with the
other hand. This is depicted in Figures
6-7A and 6-7B.

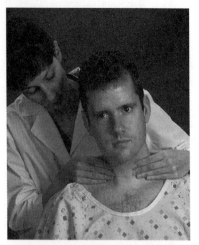

A. Posterior Approach

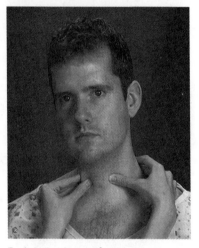

B. Anterior Approach

Figure 6-7   Examination of the Thyroid
Gland

It is important to be aware of the older
adult's safety and security needs during
this procedure. Placing fingers on an individual's throat might make some persons
anxious. Explanation of the procedure in
a calm, soothing, step-by-step fashion is
likely to reduce a client's fear. If the older
adult has trouble swallowing, repeated
sips of water may cause aspiration. Proceed slowly.

If the thyroid gland is found to be enlarged, the nurse should auscultate for **bruits,** blowing or swishing noises, from the increased vascularity associated with an enlarged thyroid. Use the bell of the stethoscope to auscultate.

Upon inspection, lymph nodes in the head and neck region should not be visible. The lymphatic vessels comprise a remarkable filtering system throughout the body. Their location in the head and neck area is indicated in Figure 6-3. Palpation of the lymph nodes is depicted in Figures 6-8A through 6-8I.

Enlarged, hard, or tender nodes can indicate a variety of pathologies, including tuberculosis, abdominal or thoracic malignancies, streptococcal or bacterial infections, and AIDS.

Summary

Assessment of the head and neck of an older adult can reap findings indicative of pathological conditions warranting nursing intervention. Elicit subjective data on history of headaches, sinus infections, hypertension, ocular problems, injury, or accidents. Obtain objective data from

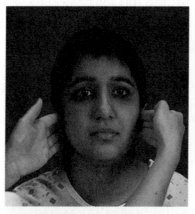

A. Preauricular

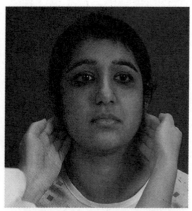

B. Postauricular

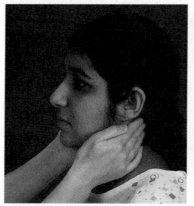

C. Occipital

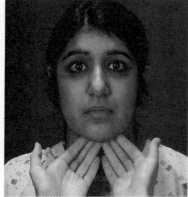

D. Submental

Figure 6-8 Palpation of Lymph Nodes

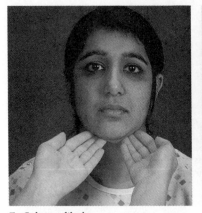

E. Submandibular

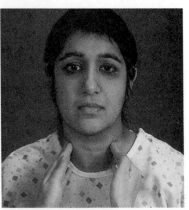

F. Anterior Cervical Chain

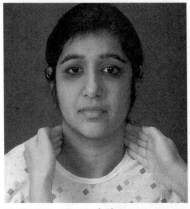

G. Posterior Cervical Chain

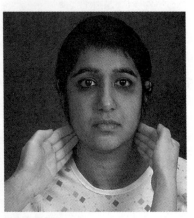

H. Tonsillar

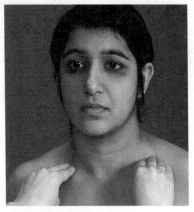

I. Supraclavicular

inspection and palpation of the head, scalp, face, mandible, neck, thyroid gland, and lymph glands. Consider environmental, psychosocial factors, medical diagnoses, and history along with associated lab tests to formulate a care plan.

References

Burke, M., & Walsh, M. (1997). *Gerontologic nursing: Wholistic care of the older adult.* St. Louis: Mosby.

Cauthorne-Burnette, T., & Zator Estes, M. (1998). *Clinical companion for health assessment and physical examination.* Albany: Delmar Publishers.

Zator Estes, M. (1998). *Health assessment & physical examination.* Albany: Delmar Publishers.

7

Sensory Assessment

Key Terms

air conduction
aqueous humor
arcus senilis
blepharitis
blepharospasm
bone conduction
canker sore
cataracts
cerumen
chancre
conjuntivitis
dysphagia
dysphasia
ectropion
edentulous
entropion
exophthalmos
fovea centralis
gingivitis
glaucoma
Hirschberg test
hordeolum
IOP (intraocular pressure)
iris
lacrimal gland
leukoplakia
miotic
mydriatic
myopia
myxedema
nystagmus
ophthalmoscope
ophthalmologist
optometrist
otoscope
presbycusis
presbyopia
pterygium
ptosis
red reflex
Rinne test
Snellen chart
tonometry
tragus
uvula
Weber test
xanthelasma

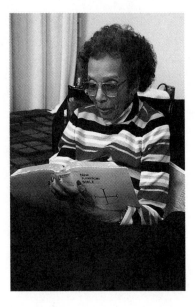

TIPS FROM THE EXPERTS

Eyes, ears, nose, and throat examination places the nurse directly in the client's "space." Anxiety, dementia, or signs of confusion must be recognized so that a calm, gentle, unrushed approach is maintained.

The senses and related body organs permit the older person to experience the world. When any one of the senses—sight, hearing, smelling, or taste—is affected, the older person's experience of the her or his surroundings is muted or altered. This alteration, in turn, has physiological, interpersonal, psychosocial, and sometimes spiritual repercussions, which may have a negative influence on an older person's life. Sensory alterations may be misperceived as confusion or dementia. The gerontological nurse is in a prime position to screen for and assist in correction of sensory problems.

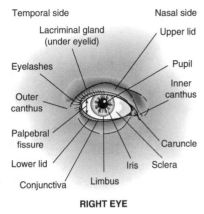

Figure 7-1   External View of the Eye

Anatomy and Physiology

Familiarity with anatomical structures of the eye, ear, nose, mouth, and throat are necessary to begin to understand any changes.

Figures 7-1 through 7-8 show anatomical landmarks.

Sensory Age-Related Changes

Tables 7-1, 7-2, and 7-3 summarize "normal" age-related changes in senses.

Pertinent Aspects of the Health History

Important background information on past and present sensory issues must be ascertained to establish an effective plan of care. History of **glaucoma, cataracts, conjunctivitis,** ear infections, and stroke with resultant **dysphagia** and **dysphasia** are all critical to subsequent examination. It is important to note any assistive devices such as eyeglasses, hearing aides, and dentures used to enhance sensory perception. Dates of the last eye, ear, and dental exams confirm appropriate update and preventive care.

Nasal passages are critical to the mechanics of breathing and tasting. Solicit information on history of polyps, sinus infection, septal deviation, and allergic rhinitis. Frequency of upper respiratory infections (URIs) should be noted. Use of tobacco, snuff, and chewing tobacco may contribute to otolaryngeal and respiratory

Table 7-1   Summary of Age-Related Vision Changes

Eyes/vision
   graying of eyebrows and eye-
     lashes
   atrophy of skin surrounding eyes
   ↓ corneal sensitivity
   ↓ corneal reflex
   tendency for "dry eyes": ↓ tear se-
     cretion
   arcus senilis: cloudy ring around
     the iris
   ↓ pigment in iris
   presbyopia: ↓ ability to focus, ac-
     commodate
   ↓ lens flexibility, yellowing
   difficulty discriminating blue-green
     colors (↓ short wavelength dis-
     crimination)
   ↓ pupillary size and ↓ response to
     light/dark
   ↓ tolerance to glare
   some ↓ in peripheral vision

Adapted from Matteson, M., McConnell, E.S., & Linton, A.D. (1997). *Gerontological nursing: Concepts and practice.* Philadelphia: W. B. Saunders.

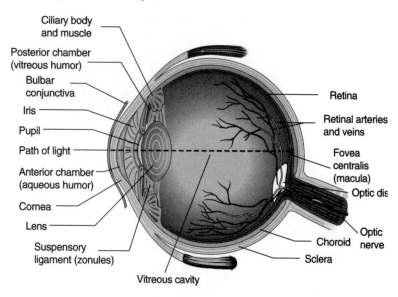

Figure 7-2   Lateral Cross-Section of the Interior Eye

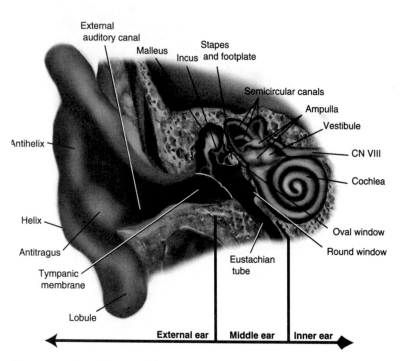

Figure 7-3   Cross-Section of the Ear

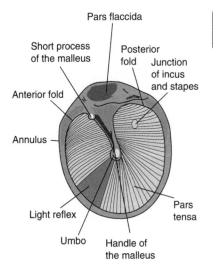

Figure 7-4 Tympanic Membrane

Table 7-2 Summary of Age-Related Hearing Changes

Ears/hearing
atrophy of external ears, wrinkling
dryness and itching of external
ears
coarser ear hair
hardening of **cerumen** (ear wax)
thickening of eardrum
↓ equilibrium due to vestibular
changes
presbycusis: ↓ hearing acuity
- difficulty hearing high frequencies
- difficulty tolerating loud
noises and background noises
- symptoms are bilateral
↓ ability to discern consonants
("g", "s", "f", etc. create high-frequency sounds)

Adapted from Matteson, M. McConnell,
E.S., & Linton, A.D. (1997). *Gerontological nursing: Concepts and practice.*
Philadelphia: W. B. Saunders.

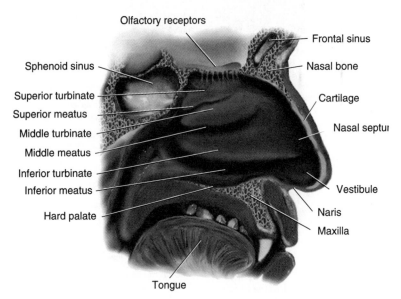

Figure 7-5 Lateral Cross-Section of the Nose

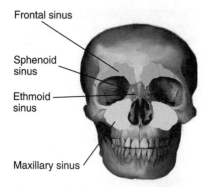

Frontal sinus

Sphenoid sinus

Ethmoid sinus

Maxillary sinus

Figure 7-6 Location of the Sinuses (Sphenoid sinuses are directly behind ethmoid sinuses)

abnormalities. Surgical procedures such as cataract extraction, retinal repair, tumor removal or cosmetic surgery should be documented.

The nurse may not have access to sensory measurement equipment listed above. Foregoing some aspects of assessment may be necessary yet compensated by referral to the indicated health care team member or by obtaining recent examination findings, which should be noted appropriately.

Eye Assessment

Visual acuity, visual fields, internal and external eye structures, movement and light

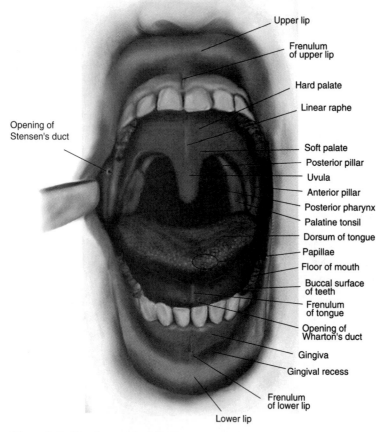

Upper lip

Frenulum of upper lip

Hard palate

Linear raphe

Opening of Stensen's duct

Soft palate

Posterior pillar

Uvula

Anterior pillar

Posterior pharynx

Palatine tonsil

Dorsum of tongue

Papillae

Floor of mouth

Buccal surface of teeth

Frenulum of tongue

Opening of Wharton's duct

Gingiva

Gingival recess

Frenulum of lower lip

Lower lip

Figure 7-7 Structures of the Mouth

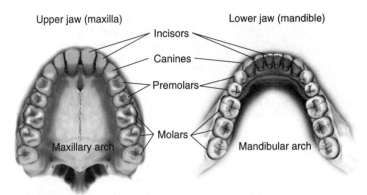

Upper jaw (maxilla)
Lower jaw (mandible)
Incisors
Canines
Premolars
Maxillary arch
Molars
Mandibular arch

Figure 7-8   Permanent Teeth

Table 7-3   Summary of Age-Related Changes in Taste, Smell, and Touch

Taste, Smell, and Touch:
↓ in taste buds (gradual)
atrophy of olfactory bulbs
changes in taste and smell as "age-related" is controversial and inconclusive
↓ sensitivity to vibration
pain perception: no conclusive evidence of age as a predictor of cutaneous and deep pain

Adapted from Matteson, M., McConnell, E.S., & Linton, A.D. (1997). *Gerontological nursing: Concepts and practice*. Philadelphia: W. B. Saunders.

✓ **NURSING CHECKLIST**

General Approach to Eyes, Ears, Nose, Mouth, and Throat Assessment

• Explain the assessment techniques that you will be using.
• Ensure that the light in the room provides sufficient brightness to allow adequate observation of the patient.
• Place the patient in an upright, sitting position on the examination table.
• Always use a systematic approach and compare right and left eyes and ears as well as right and left sides of the nose, sinuses, mouth, and throat.

reflex, and anterior and posterior structures of the eyes are examined in a full eye examination. The depth of the eye exam is contingent upon availability of equipment, skillfulness of the clinician, and cooperation of the client.

Distance Vision

Visual acuity tests CNII (second cranial nerve). Use the **Snellen chart**. The client should stand 20 feet away from the chart. With eyeglasses removed, the occluder is applied to one eye. Request that the client read as many lines on the chart as possi-

ble. Make a notation of the number at the end of the last line the client is able to read. If the client is unable to read the largest print at 20 feet, ask him or her to move closer and note the number of feet from the chart. Repeat this procedure with the opposite eye and also with glasses on (note uncorrected and corrected vision results). 20/20 vision is considered normal visual acuity. It is not uncommon to find **myopia** (nearsightedness) or visual acuity different for each eye. Chronic diseases are known to affect eyesight. These include

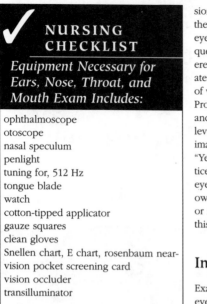

✔ **NURSING CHECKLIST**

Equipment Necessary for Ears, Nose, Throat, and Mouth Exam Includes:

ophthalmoscope
otoscope
nasal speculum
penlight
tuning for, 512 Hz
tongue blade
watch
cotton-tipped applicator
gauze squares
clean gloves
Snellen chart, E chart, rosenbaum near-vision pocket screening card
vision occluder
transilluminator

diabetes, renal disease, hypertension, and atherosclerosis, to name a few.

Near Vision and Color Vision

Presbyopia (farsightedness) is a very common finding in people over 40 years old. It is considered part of the natural aging process. Test for farsightedness by using a Rosenbaum card or appropriate reading material. Request that the client sit comfortably and read the card at 14 inches from the face. The client reads the smallest possible line if using a Rosenbaum card. Use of other reading material will yield helpful results.

Ask the client to identify the six primary colors on the Snellen chart. Presence of **macular degeneration**, nutritional deficiency, and heredity affect color identification. Difficulty in distinguishing blues from greens is considered within the parameters of "normal aging."

Visual Fields

Visual fields test assesses CNII (second cranial nerve) and degree of peripheral vi-

sion. While sitting 2 to 3 feet opposite from the client, ask the client to cover her right eye. Similarly, you cover your left eye. Request that the client focus on your uncovered eye. Stretch out your free hand. Situate your hand at you and your client's field of vision at nose level. Move your fingers. Proceed to temporal, superior, inferior, and oblique angles, moving fingers at each level. These positions assimilate four imaginary quadrants. Ask the client to say "Yes" when movement of fingers is noticed. Repeat this procedure with the other eye. Match the client's response to your own. Problems such as stroke, glaucoma, or retinal detachment will affect results of this test.

Inspection of External Eyes

Examine for abnormal drooping of the eyelids, exudate from the eyes, redness, or asymmetry. Inspect eyelashes and eyebrows for distribution of hair; uneven distribution may indicate an endocrine disorder.

Ask the client to follow your finger. Start about 12 inches from the nose of the client, and move your finger downward, slowly. Look for symmetrical movement and blinking of the eyes. Observe sclera, which should appear white. Next, ask the client to raise eyelids. Again, look for symmetry of movement, influenced by CNIII (cranial nerve III). The eyelids should cover the top curve of the iris. Excessive drooping, called **ptosis**, is shown in Figure 7-9.

Common pathological findings of the eye are described in Table 7-4.

Assessment of Lacrimal Apparatus

Inspect the outside of the **lacrimal gland**, at the upper eyelid. Note any redness, swelling, and puffiness of the eyelid, exudate, or tearing. Compare both eyes. Tenderness, exudate, or redness should not be present. Inflammation of the lacrimal gland suggests an obstruction or infection.

Don gloves and palpate the lacrimal

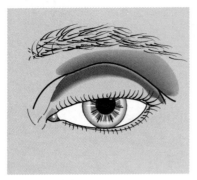

Figure 7-9 Ptosis

gland at the inner canthus. Slight tearing is within normal limits.

Extraocular Muscle Function

Eye movement is coordinated and controlled by six muscles (see Figure 7-10). It is assessed employing three tests: corneal light reflex, cover/uncover test, and cardinal fields of gaze (cranial nerves III, IV, and VI).

Corneal Light Reflex (Hirschberg Test)

While the client looks straight ahead, shine a penlight about 14 inches from the corneas. The reflected light should shine at the center of each cornea, demonstrating equivalent muscle response. Asymmetrical response is shown in Figure 7-11. Neurological conditions may be the cause of asymmetrical muscle response.

Cover/Uncover Test

As the client looks straight ahead at a distant object, place the occluder over the eye for several seconds. Observe the uncovered eye for movement. Then remove the occluder. Observe the newly uncovered eye for movement Repeat this procedure by having the client focus on an object held close to the eye. Test the opposite eye. Coordinated movement is considered normal. Mild muscle weakness may cause misalignment of the eyes and drifting. **Nys-**

Table 7-4 Common Pathological Findings of the Eye
Ptosis: excessive drooping of the eyelid • mechanical—from lesions, adipose tissue, or edema • myogenic—from muscular disorders (such as multiple sclerosis) • neurogenic—from neurological disorders (such as paralysis, stroke, neuronal disruption) **Lagophthalmos:** incomplete closing of lid **Dacryoadenitis:** pain in the eye at upper lateral aspect at site of lacrimal gland **Exophthalmos:** lid retraction and eye protrusion **Blepharospasm:** contractions of orbicularis oculi muscle (due to CNVII lesions, eye irritation, or fatigue or stress) **Hordeolum:** sty, usually found around the lid **Blepharitis:** inflammation of one or both lids, often due to infection or irritation **Xanthelasma:** yellow plaques on lids, which may suggest hypercholesteremia

tagmus (rhythmic, involuntary eye movement) should not be present.

Cardinal Fields of Gaze

While the client faces the nurse, she or he is instructed to follow an object or the nurse's finger at six points (see Figure 7-12).

Return to the midline after moving through each of the six fields and note eye movement, which should be smooth and coordinated. As the eyes meet the midline, move the object about 6 inches from the client's nose. Eyes should converge.

Movement deviations reflect varied degrees of nerve damage:

- eye is unable to move outward: CN VI
- eye cannot move downward and inward: CN IV
- variations in movement: CN III

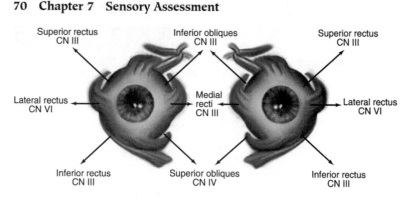

Figure 7-10   Direction of Movement of Extaocular Muscles

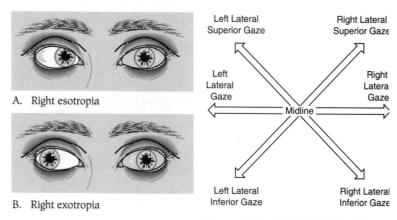

A. Right esotropia

B. Right exotropia

Figure 7-11 Asymmetrical Corneal Light Reflex

Figure 7-12   Cardinal Fields of Gaze

Fracture or injury to the orbit may result in some form of cranial nerve damage. In addition, botulism, herpes zoster, syphilis, or vitamin deficiency (thiamin especially) may lead to defects in eye movements.

Head injury and increased intracranial pressure influence eye movement. The location and severity of head trauma influences the degree of muscle and nerve damage of the eyes:

- increased intracranial pressure: optic muscle paralysis
- midbrain trauma, tumors: vertical gaze deviation
- cerebral cortex, motor center damage: horizontal gaze deviation

- lesion in the pons: skew deviation (one eye up, one eye down)
- brainstem, visual pathway trauma: nystagmus

Anterior Structures of the Eye

Assess the conjunctiva by gently parting the lid margins. As the client looks up and down, note the bulbar conjunctiva for redness, exudate, swelling, or foreign bodies. The conjunctiva should appear clear white with small blood vessels spread throughout. Sticky exudate and lid swelling may suggest bacterial conjunctivitis, which is best treated with antibiotic therapy.

Pterygium is a common finding. This is a triangular thickening on the nasal side of the conjunctiva (refer to Figure 7-13).

Subconjunctival hemorrhage, a painless reddish appearance of the bulbar conjunctiva, may be the result of increased pressure from hypertension, coughing, sneezing, Valsalva maneuver (bearing down), or anticoagulant therapy. This finding warrants investigation into the cause of the pressure.

Sclera should appear white upon inspection. In dark-skinned individuals specks of melanin may be present. Jaundice (yellow sclera) or a blue color (thinning of the sclera) are abnormal findings warranting diagnostic lab testing for blood abnormalities.

Examine the cornea by inspection. Flash a penlight directly on the cornea. The surface of the cornea should appear smooth, shiny, and free from ulceration. A cloudy cornea may indicate glaucoma, which is caused by insufficient drainage from the **aqueous humor**. **IOP (intraoccular pressure)** increases, causing damages to the eye's ability to discern objects mid-peripherally and eventually, centrally. **Tonometry** measures eye pressure and is a lifesaving intervention that preserves an older person's vision. Tonometry readings should range between 13 and 22. The most common and effective treatment is pharmacological. Ophthalmic drops such as timolol maleate reduce pressure and allow for proper drainage through the canal of Schlemm. As with any medication, side effects of eye drops must be monitored and reinforced through client teaching.

In light-eyed individuals it is common to find **arcus senilis**, a grayish ring or band inside the limbus. This is not a pathological finding but a result of breakdown of the peripheral cornea. In contrast, herpes simplex virus can cause a branch-like surface on the cornea, accompanied by pain, discomfort, and blurred vision. Refer to an **ophthalmologist**.

NURSING TIP

Collaboration with the ophthalmologist, who specializes in disorders of the eye, is necessary for treatment of glaucoma, cataracts, retinal detachment, or diabetic retinopathy. Do not confuse the ophthalmologist with the optometrist. The former is able to perform surgery. The optometrist tests for visual acuity and prescribes glasses accordingly.

Using a penlight, inspect the **iris**. Note color, smoothness, and vascularity. Normally, the iris is smooth and its color is distributed evenly. Unevenness or raised pigmented areas of the iris may indicate melanoma or trauma and warrant referral.

Testing the pupils serves three assessment purposes:

- determines the speed of reaction to light stimulus
- determines the accommodation and ability to focus
- sheds insight into neurological pathologies

While the client is in a darkened room, take notice of pupillary shape and size (in millimeters). In a sweeping motion, move the light from the side to the center of the pupil and back to the side. Observe the reaction, noting the size and speed of response. Examine the other eye.

To test for accommodation, ask the client to focus on a distant object. Then ask the client to focus on your pen, held

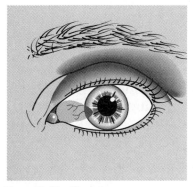

Figure 7-13   Pterygium

12 centimeters from the client's nose. Observe the pupils for size and ability to converge. The ability to focus far to near is a key skill used in driving and thus mandates that the nurse pay special attention to the findings. Similarly, pupillary response holds implications for night driving, which requires the eyes to adjust and regulate the entry of light.

The pupillary size ranges from 2 to 6 millimeters. Response should be quick and equal. Ability for accommodation, far to near, measures CN III. A **miotic** response (pupil 2 millimeters in diameter) or **mydriatic** response (> 6 millimeters) suggests medications such as sympathomimetics or CN III paralysis from carotid artery insufficiency. An irregularly shaped pupil may indicate removal of a cataract or iridectomy. Brain lesion or optic nerve damage causes a vacillating response to light. Table 7-5 shows variations in pupillary response.

The lens rests behind the pupil. Shine a penlight on the pupil. The lens should appear clear/transparent. A pearly gray appearance indicates a cataract. Cataract surgery is the most frequently performed surgery in older people. It is a simple yet skilled surgical procedure allowing the "cloud of darkness" to be removed from the eyes. Cataract removal and replacement with a synthetic lens allow individuals to enjoy the detail and beauty the environment offers. Chronological age should not be a reason for not performing cataract surgery.

Posterior Structures of the Eye

An ophthalmoscope is necessary to examine the posterior eye structure. Not all gerontological nurses have access to or the skill to perform this exam. Still, the procedure is described.

Retinal Structures

A fundoscopic assessment measuring CN II is conducted in a darkened room with eyeglasses removed.

The first step is attainment of the **red reflex**. While the client is focusing on a far object, shine the light of the ophthalmoscope (set at O lens) at a 15 degree angle into the client's pupil. Remain about 12 inches from the client. The light reflects off the retina. The diopter wheel should be moved from 0 to the +, or black, numbers to focus on ocular structures. Get close to the client—about an inch—from the client's eye. Move the −, or red, numbers to visualize more posterior structures. View the optic disc toward the nasal side of the retina. See Figures 7-14 and 7-15.

Look at the retina for color and lesions. Note and describe the optic disc—color, shape, size, and margins. The diameter of the optic disc is used to describe the distance from other noted points of abnormal findings. Perform on both eyes. Carefully review Table 7-6 for retinal color.

The optic disc should appear pinkish with a yellow-white center (physiologic cup). Cup to disc diameter is about 1:3. Four major vascular branches should be evident. Again, examine Figure 7-2. As light reflects off arterioles, it appears shiny. Some abnormal findings are listed in Table 7-7.

Macula

The macula is viewed by moving the ophthalmoscope from the optic disc over about 2 disc diameters. The macula is not easily discerned because it is not sharply demarcated. The **fovea centralis** is located central to the macula and is very sensitive to light. While a healthy macula will appear darker, the fovea centralis will appear like a point with a reflective center. Findings of macular degeneration include a blurry border of the macula and pigmented or hole-like center. Macular degeneration is accompanied by loss of central vision. Early laser treatment may improve the condition.

Assessment of the Ears

Figures 7–3 and 7–4 (pages 64 and 65) depict the anatomy of the ear. There are three major components of ear assessment: voice-whisper test, tuning fork test, and otoscopic assessment. How the individual communicates is a key issue in de-

Table 7-5 Pupil Abnormalities

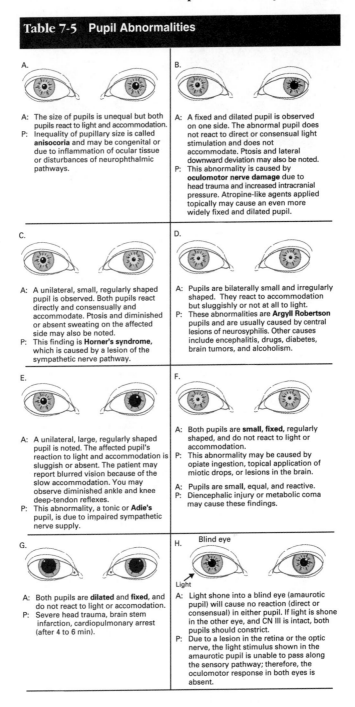

A.

A: The size of pupils is unequal but both pupils react to light and accommodation.

P: Inequality of pupillary size is called **anisocoria** and may be congenital or due to inflammation of ocular tissue or disturbances of neurophthalmic pathways.

B.

A: A fixed and dilated pupil is observed on one side. The abnormal pupil does not react to direct or consensual light stimulation and does not accommodate. Ptosis and lateral downward deviation may also be noted.

P: This abnormality is caused by **oculomotor nerve damage** due to head trauma and increased intracranial pressure. Atropine-like agents applied topically may cause an even more widely fixed and dilated pupil.

C.

A: A unilateral, small, regularly shaped pupil is observed. Both pupils react directly and consensually and accommodate. Ptosis and diminished or absent sweating on the affected side may also be noted.

P: This finding is **Horner's syndrome,** which is caused by a lesion of the sympathetic nerve pathway.

D.

A: Pupils are bilaterally small and irregularly shaped. They react to accommodation but sluggishly or not at all to light.

P: These abnormalities are **Argyll Robertson** pupils and are usually caused by central lesions of neurosyphilis. Other causes include encephalitis, drugs, diabetes, brain tumors, and alcoholism.

E.

A: A unilateral, large, regularly shaped pupil is noted. The affected pupil's reaction to light and accommodation is sluggish or absent. The patient may report blurred vision because of the slow accommodation. You may observe diminished ankle and knee deep-tendon reflexes.

P: This abnormality, a tonic or **Adie's** pupil, is due to impaired sympathetic nerve supply.

F.

A: Both pupils are **small, fixed,** regularly shaped, and do not react to light or accommodation.

P: This abnormality may be caused by opiate ingestion, topical application of miotic drops, or lesions in the brain.

A: Pupils are small, equal, and reactive.

P: Diencephalic injury or metabolic coma may cause these findings.

G.

A: Both pupils are **dilated** and **fixed,** and do not react to light or accomodation.

P: Severe head trauma, brain stem infarction, cardiopulmonary arrest (after 4 to 6 min).

H. Blind eye

Light

A: Light shone into a blind eye (amaurotic pupil) will cause no reaction (direct or consensual) in either pupil. If light is shone in the other eye, and CN III is intact, both pupils should constrict.

P: Due to a lesion in the retina or the optic nerve, the light stimulus shown in the amaurotic pupil is unable to pass along the sensory pathway; therefore, the oculomotor response in both eyes is absent.

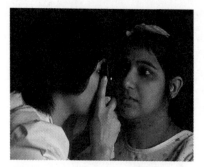

Figure 7-14   Examining Retinal Structures: Funduscopic Examination

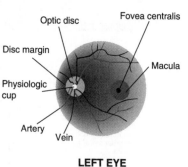

LEFT EYE

Figure 7-15   Optic Disk

termining hearing. Misinterpretation, paranoia, or inappropriate responses may indicate inability to hear clearly. In addition, how older people cope with hearing loss is also an important factor in compensating.

Voice-Whisper Test

Although it is rudimentary, the voice-whisper test is useful to discern obvious hearing problems.

Stand about 2 feet from the client, facing each other. To test the left ear, ask the client to block the right ear. Stand on the left side of the client. Instruct the client to repeat the sentence you will say. Camouflage your mouth with your hand (kept flat). Whisper the sentence. Repeat this procedure with the right ear. The client should be able to repeat the sentence. If not, some form of hearing loss probably exits.

Tuning fork tests

The **Weber** and **Rinne tests** distinguish conductive from sensorineural hearing loss. Air conduction versus bone conduction is tested. Carefully explain the procedure and feelings of vibration to the older

Table 7-6 Retinal Color Variations	
FINDINGS	**CHARACTERISTICS**
Light-skinned individuals	Retina appears a lighter red-orange color
	Tessellated appearance of the fundi (pigment does not obscure the choroid vessels)
Dark-skinned individuals	Fundi appear darker in color; grayish purple to brownish (from increased pigment in the choroid and retina)
	No tessellated appearance
	Choroidal vessels usually obscured
Aging individuals	Vessels are straighter and narrower
	Choroidal vessels are easily visualized
	Retinal pigment epithelium atrophies and causes the retinal color to become paler

Table 7-7 Some Abnormal Findings in the Retinal Structures

Findings	Possible Causes
Pale optic disc	atrophy from (intracranial pressure)
Papillitis (disc edema)	optic neuritis; (intracranial pressure)
Roth spots (retinal hemorrhages)	severe hypertension, blockage in central retinal vein, infective endocarditis
Deeper retinal hemorrhages	diabetes mellitus
Microaneurysms (small red dots) in macular areas of the retina	diabetic retinopathy
Fluffy white areas on retina	nerve fiber infarcts from diabetic retinopathy and hypertension
Detached retina: no red reflex pearly gray, raised	cataract surgery, trauma, and myopia

Adapted from Cauthorne-Burnette, T., & Estes, M. (1998). *Clinical companion for health assessment and physical examination*. Albany: Delmar/ITP Publishers.

person, who may not be comfortable with these sensations.

Weber Test

Activate the tuning fork by striking it on the outer border of the palm. As it is vibrating, place the stem on either the middle of the client's forehead or middle of the top of the head. See Figure 7–16.

Ask the client where the sound is heard, either centrally or on one side. Normal findings comprise hearing the sound centrally or "in the middle." Normal findings are known as a "negative" Weber test. Abnormal findings are summarized in Table 7-8.

Rinne Test

Strike the tuning fork. Place the stem on the right mastoid process to assess **bone conduction.** See Figure 7-17A. Ask the client to tell you whether the sound is heard. If yes, ask the client to state when the sound stops.

Moving the tuning fork at the right auditory meatus after the client tells you the sound has stopped tests **air conduction.** See Figure 7-17(B). Ask if the sound is still heard and note the length of time the client hears the sounds.

Test the left ear. Sound is heard twice as long by way of the external auditory canal (air conduction) than by bone conduction by way of the mastoid process.

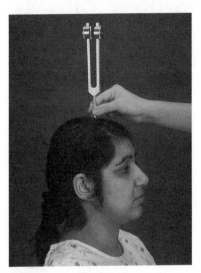

Figure 7-16 Weber Test

If sound is heard longer through bone, conductive hearing loss due to damage, diseases, or obstruction of the outer or middle ear is suspected.

External Ear

Inspect the external ears for position, size, shape, inflammation, and lesions. Note cerumen. Instead of moist brown cerumen, it is not uncommon to find dry, hard,

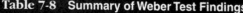

Table 7-8   Summary of Weber Test Findings

Findings	Possible disorder
Client hears sound "in the middle":	none likely
Client hears sound on left side or right side:	The side where the sound is heard is likely to have conductive hearing loss • Middle ear disorder • Impacted cerumen • Perforated tympanic membrane
Client hears sound in unimpaired ear (sensorineural hearing loss):	Nerve damage in impaired ear; inner ear, auditory nerve, or brain damage; ototoxicity

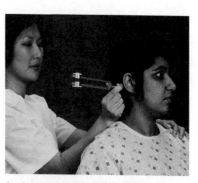

A. Assessing Bone Conduction

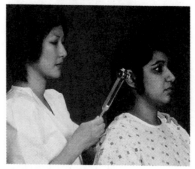

B. Assessing Air Conduction

Figure 7-17   Rinne Test

and large accumulations in the ear canal of the older client. Refer to Table 7-2 (page 65) for age-related changes to the ear. Abnormal findings include any type of

drainage, nodules, or swelling, which warrants referral to a specialist.

Palpate the auricle, mastoid tip, and **tragus** with the index and middle fingers. Pain and tenderness comprise abnormal findings suggesting possible mastoiditis or otitis externa.

Otoscopic Assessment

The otoscope is used to view the tympanic membrane. Find the largest speculum attachment, which will fit the ear canal. Comfortably hold the otoscope with the head down. (See Figure 7-18).

Gently pull the ear upward and backward to straighten the canal. If cerumen is present, remove it by irrigating gently.

Advance the speculum into the canal. Observe for redness, lesions, or inflammation. When fully advanced, the tympanic membrane should be visible. It should appear pearly to dull gray. Landmarks should be noted: the handle of the malleus, umbo, and light reflex. Hard, dark brown cerumen may indicate canal impaction. Excessive redness and absent light reflex suggest otitis media. A darkened "hole" in the tympanic membrane or patches indicates a perforation or scarring from old perforations.

Assessment of the Nose

Observe for any masses, lesions, bleeding, swelling, or apparent deviation. Test for

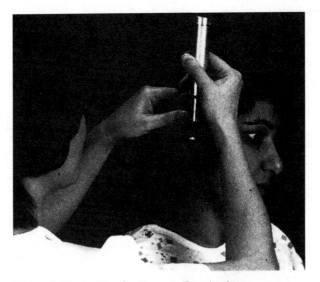

Figure 7-18   Position for Otoscope Examination

patency by asking the client to breathe while blocking one nostril. Repeat for opposite nostril. Deviated septum, polyps, allergy, or infection are possible causes of difficulty.

Internal inspection of the nasal passages requires using the otoscope. Select a short, wide speculum. Examine one nasal passage at a time for status of mucous membranes, drainage, bleeding, or perforation. No swelling or bleeding should be found. The nasal septum should be positioned approximately midline. Edema, redness, swelling, or clear drainage may indicate allergies and rhinitis. Purulent drainage other than clear and red mucous membranes either unilaterally or bilaterally may suggest bacterial infection, overuse of nasal spray, or drug use such as cocaine.

Sinuses are inspected and palpated to rule out possible infection. Irritations or infections in the sinus passages are not only painful but also interfere with effective breathing.

Inspect for swelling around the nose and eyes. None should be present. Palpate the frontal and maxillary sinuses as shown in Figure 7-19 A & B. The client should feel no pain.

Use the middle finger of the dominant hand to directly percuss under the bony area of the upper orbits. Note the sound. With the thumbs, gently press the area under the infraorbital ridges.

Note any pain. Directly percuss the same area and note the sound. Sinuses should have a resonant sound because they are air-filled. Dull sounds indicate fluid-filled tissue, possibly because of infection or allergy.

Assessment of the Mouth and Throat

The mouth, throat, and teeth are important vehicles for communication and expression. In addition, they help individuals enjoy food. A healthy oral cavity is important for a positive body image and for functionality.

Dentures should be removed. Gloves are donned. A penlight or ample light is used for adequate visualization.

Note the client's breath. Foul-smelling breath may indicate poor oral hygiene, tooth or gum disease, or sinus infection. Fruity breath is associated with malnutrition or diabetic ketoacidosis. Ammonia

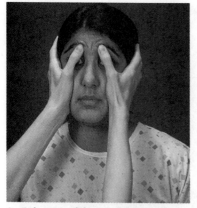

A. Palpation of the Frontal Sinuses

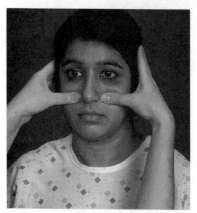

B. Palpation of Maxillary Sinuses

Figure 7-19   Palpation of the Sinuses

breath is associated with uremia and end-stage renal failure.

Observe the lips, which should appear pink, moist, and without lesions or swelling. Palpate the upper and lower lips by gently pulling them down or up. The tone of the lips should be somewhat firm and without lesions, warts, cold sores, or ulcers. Such abnormal findings mandate referral to a dentist. Distinguish between simple cold sores (herpes simplex lesions) and **chancre** (round painless lesion with central ulceration found in clients with syphilis). **Leukoplakia** (white patches on the lips) are caused by tobacco or excessive alcohol use. Cyanosis of the lips indi-

cates insufficient oxygen in the blood and poor circulation.

Inspect the position of the tongue, which should be midline in the mouth. It should appear pink, moist, and rough. The underside of the tongue should have ample blood vessels and no lesions or open areas. Ask the client to stick out the tongue (CN XII). Hydration, texture, and symmetry are noted. Ask the client to move the tongue left and right, up and down. Palpate the tongue through the cheek when the client moves the tongue left and right. Note the strength.

Inspect the ventral side of the tongue by grasping the tongue with a gauze pad and gently moving it side to side. The frenulum ("divider") of the tongue should appear smooth. Wharton's ducts should appear patent.

An enlarged tongue may suggest **myxedema**, cellulitis of the neck, hematoma, or abscess. A red, smooth tongue may suggest B-12, iron, or niacin deficiencies. "Thrush" (candidiasis) is a thick white coating on the tongue associated with antibiotic therapy, chemotherapy, immune system disorders, or substance abuse, all of which upset the natural oral flora.

Painful small white lesions or **canker sores** are caused by stress, food allergy, oral trauma, or extreme fatigue. Prolonged antibiotic therapy can result in yellow, black, or brown coloring to the tongue with a hairy appearance (hairy leukoplakia). Lesions on the tongue are associated with lingual cancers. A dry, furrowed tongue with more than one longitudinal demarcation, along with lack of saliva accumulation in the floor of the mouth, suggests severe dehydration.

The buccal mucosa is examined by using a tongue depressor and penlight and inspecting the inner cheeks and Stensen's ducts. African Americans have a bluish hue to the buccal mucosa whereas Caucasians have pink mucosa. Lesions, dryness, or ulceration are abnormal findings. Pale mucosa paired with excessive dry mouth suggests vasoconstriction and severe dehydration.

Gums should appear red-pink without

pocketing or separation from the teeth. Swelling and bleeding are abnormal findings caused by poor oral hygiene, **gingivitis**, poor denture fit, or medication use such as phenytoin. Vitamin C can enhance gum health and healing.

Many older people are **edentulous**, (they have no teeth). Modern dentistry has aggressively promoted preventive measures in tooth and gum preservation, which will impact current baby boomers and their children more so than the current generation of older people. An adult has thirty-two teeth. Because of trauma, bruxism (grinding of teeth), decay, neglect, or cosmetic reasons more or less than thirty-two teeth may be noted. Ineffective chewing from painful teeth or lack of teeth influences the nutrition of older people. See Chapter 14 on Nutritional Assessment.

Observe the hard and soft palates by viewing with a penlight. The client will need to open the mouth wide. The soft palate is closer to the throat whereas the hard palate is closer to the front teeth. The palate should appear arched, pink, and smooth, with no lesions or ulcerations. Any erosion of the palate should be noted.

Inspect the throat by depressing the middle of the tongue and viewing with a penlight. Ask the client to say "ah," which opens the passage. Note tonsils and **uvula**; swelling, redness, or lesions are abnormal. Depress the posterior third of the tongue and note gag reflex (CN IX and X). The gag reflex is sometimes sluggish in some older people. Note any swallowing difficulties. Infections such as pharyngitis or tumors are two possible causes of abnormal throat findings.

Generally, dental, hearing, and eye exams should be conducted every six months to a year in older adults.

Summary

Physiological changes or pathological changes in the sensory organs are responsible for alterations or potential alterations in how an older person perceives and understands the world. Gerontological nurses are able to provide the in-depth assessment, screening, and referral to maintain and restore this vital function.

References

Burke, M., & Walsh, M. (1997). *Gerontologic nursing: Wholistic care of the older adult*. St. Louis: Mosby-Year Book, Inc.

Cauthorne-Burnette, T., & Zator Estes, M. (1998). *Clinical companion for health assessment and physical examination*. Albany: Delmar/ITP Publishers.

Matteson, M., McConnell, E.S., & Linton, A.D. (1997). *Gerontological nursing: Concepts and practice*. Philadelphia: W. B. Saunders.

✓ NURSING CHECKLIST

Preparing for the Assessment of the Mouth and Throat

- If the patient is wearing dentures or removable orthodontia, ask that they be removed before the assessment begins.
- Use gloves and a good light source, such as a penlight, for optimum visualization of the oral cavity and pharynx.

8

Respiratory Assessment

Key Terms

adventitious breath sounds
alveoli
Angle of Louis
apnea
bronchial tubes
bronchophony
bronchovesicular sounds
Cheyne-Stokes breathing
costal angle
crackles
crepitus
egophony
Kussmaul's breathing
kyphosis
lungs
manubrium
pleural friction rub
scapula
sternum
tactile fremitus
thorax
trachea
vertebra prominens
vesicular sounds
wheezes
xiphoid process

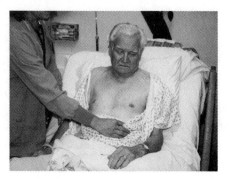

TIPS FROM THE EXPERTS

When locating skeletal landmarks on older adults, be gentle. Because of osteoporosis or less flexible bones, the nurse may accidentally injure the older adult or create unnecessary discomfort. When in doubt, ask the older adult if the palpation hurts.

Conducting a respiratory assessment in an older adult requires the nurse's knowledge of respiratory changes in functional and structural components related to the ability to exchange oxygen and carbon dioxide. Both normal aging, at least what we *think* is normal aging, as well as disease processes more prevalent in older adults comprise the foundation for understanding physical assessment and examination findings. Some of the studies that have determined normal or expected changes associated with aging have been conducted on older adults with existing problems as well as on older adults with less than desirable health habits, such as smokers. Thus, conclusions about normal aging are somewhat speculative.

Psychosocial, socioeconomic, and environmental factors influence respiratory health as they intertwine with health-seeking behaviors. This chapter addresses age-related changes related to respiratory health, key anatomical landmarks and definitions, steps of the respiratory assessment, and health promotion and disease prevention strategies.

Respiratory Changes in Older Adults

As people age, current research indicates that their ability to take in air, sort out the oxygen for transport in the bloodstream and dispose of carbon dioxide, through exhalation decreases. **Kyphosis**, which is the curvature of the spine giving the older adult a "hunched over" appearance, works against the lungs in the amount of air inhaled. The **thorax** shortens, contributing to increased anterior-posterior chest diameter. The diaphragm rallies to counteract the change but must fight against compression from the skeletal changes. In addition, structural obstacles to air exchange are compounded by stretched-out stiff **alveoli** cells at the base of the lungs. Although the alveoli are larger in older adults, they are less flexible. Because of the rigidity of these cells, it becomes difficult to empty air efficiently. In fact, when an older adult is forced to breathe rapidly, alveoli snap shut prematurely. Thus, it be-

comes challenging for the older adult to compensate under the varied stressors to the body, such as extended exercise.

Besides the effects of kyphosis and alveolar changes, slightly lower hemoglobin levels in the blood diminish the amount of oxygen delivered to cells. Hemoglobin (Hgb) levels in older adults run normal to low-normal values (Matteson, McConnell, & Linton, 1997). Oxygen is vital and needed for inter- and intracellular reactions and metabolism. Ultimately, lower levels of oxygen affect overall tissue and organ health.

Table 8-1 provides a quick reference and summary of the major respiratory-related changes in older adults.

A review of basic terminology associated with the respiratory system is detailed in Table 8-2. Basic respiratory anatomy is shown in Figure 8-1.

Key Landmarks of the Thorax and Lungs

Identification of sites for respiratory examination and assessment is the first step to correctly performing the examination of the older adult. The thorax or thoracic cavity is the skeletal shell comprising ribs, sternum, vertebrae, and spinal column within which the lungs reside. Anteriorly, there are twelve sets of ribs divided by the **sternum** (breastbone), a three-part, flat bone. The top portion as it connects from the clavicles is called the **manubrium**, followed by the body of the sternum. The **Angle of Louis** (sternal angle) at the juncture of the second rib demarcates the two segments. The lower one-third of the sternum is called the **xiphoid process**, a cartilaginous protrusion that loses its pliability in older adults. In cardiopulmonary resuscitation, the xiphoid process is gently palpated so that the location of the palm of the hand for chest compressions is accurately placed *above, not on,* the xiphoid. The **costal angle** can be identified by bilaterally palpating the tenth anterior ribs with the index fingers, moving up to the base of the sternum. The fingers have "traced" the sides, which create the costal angle of approximately 90 degrees.

Table 8-1   Summary of Respiratory-Related Changes in Older Adults

Decreases in:
- Vital capacity (VC: amount of air exhaled after a deep breath
- Inspiratory capacity (amount of air inhaled after exhaling)
- Elasticity of alveoli (ability of alveoli to open and close with ease)
- Oxygen in the arteries (PaO_2 levels)
- Ability to compensate under low oxygen levels (hypoxia)
- Cough reflex (related to possible changes in the medulla portion of the brain; medullar changes may influence the speed with which the older adult responds to hypoxia)
- Ciliary functioning (cilia are tiny hairs in the nasal passage and lung parenchyma, normally sifting small particles and bacteria from the lungs)

Increases in:
- Residual volume (air that pockets in the lungs)
- Stiffening of ribcage (related to excessive calcium in costral cartilidge between the ribs)

Adapted from Matteson, M., McConnell, M., & Linton, A (1997). *Gerontological nursing: Concepts and practice* (2nd ed.), Chapter 8, "Age-related changes in the respiratory system," 258–264, Philadelphia: W. B. Saunders.

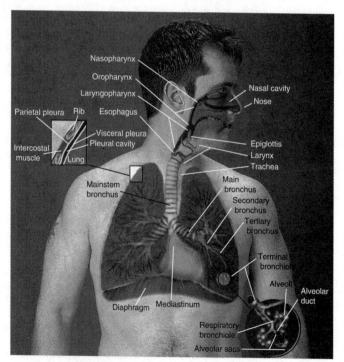

Figure 8-1   The Respiratory Tract

Table 8-2 Basic Respiratory Terminology

- *Lung parenchyma:* the composite of functional parts of the lung
- *Pharynx:* the tubular segment extending from the base of the nasal cavity to the larynx
- *Nasopharynx:* upper portion of the pharynx, above the palate
- *Oropharynx:* middle segment of the pharynx between the palate and base of the tongue
- *Laryngopharynx:* lower segment of the pharynx
- *Esophagus:* pliable muscle from pharynx to stomach; helps to carry food to stomach rather than lungs
- *Epiglottis:* a flap that covers the entrance to the larynx; functions to prevent food from being aspirated
- *Larynx:* located superior to the trachea and made up of nine cartilages; contains the vocal cords
- *Trachea:* tubular segment about 4 inches long, below larynx; branches out at the juncture called the carina, into two bronchi to left and right lungs
- *Bronchus:* branching extensions from trachea to left and right lungs; continue to divide into bronchioles
- *Cilia:* tiny hairs in the nasal and bronchial passges that move particles away from the lungs; diminished in function in older adults
- *Alveolar ducts, sacs, alveoli;* alveoli are cells in the lungs where gas exchange takes place; the alveolar ducts are tiny branches from the bronchiole that lead to sacs of the alveoli
- *Mediastinum:* contains heart and vessels, trachea and esophagus, and lymphs which separate the lungs
- *Diaphragm:* the muscle at the base of the thorax; it contracts and expands to promote respiration
- *Pleural cavity:* space sandwiched between parietal and visceral pleura
- *Visceral pleura:* portion of the moist lining against the outside of the lungs
- *Parietal pleura:* portion of the moist lining on the chest wall outside the lung to the sides of the pericardium, to the spine

Summarized from Thomas, C. L., *Taber's cyclopedic medical dictionary* (1997), Philadelphia: F. A. Davis, Estes, M. E. Z., (1998), *Health and assessment & physical examination,* Albany, NY: Delmar Publishers.

Posteriorly, the clavicles help give shape to the back and shoulders and are connected to the **scapula**, a triangular flat bone approximately spanning thoracic vertebrae T4–T7. The **vertebra prominens** is located at C7 and may be palpated if the older adult is able to flex the head forward, which is the exception in many elite older adults in their 90s.

Memorize these landmarks and refer to Figure 8-2, anterior and posterior views of the thorax. Palpate the landmarks on a colleague or willing significant other.

The **lungs** rest in the thoracic cavity and are divided into three segments on the right side and two segments on the left side (the heart inhabits the anterior middle portion of the left side of the chest). Above the top portion (or apex) of the lungs is the **trachea**, which branches out bilaterally to the **bronchial tubes**. These air-transporting tubes deliver air into the spongy matter of the lungs, down through to the alveolar ducts to the sacs, then to the alveoli, where capillaries take in oxygen and remove carbon dioxide. Figure

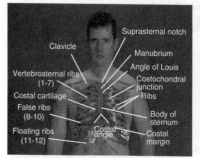

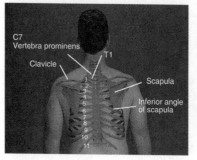

A. Anterior View

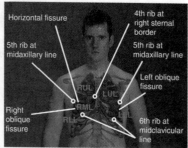

A. Anterior View

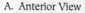

B. Posterior View

Figure 8-2 Thorax (rib number is shown on the client's right; intercostal space number is shown on the client's left.)

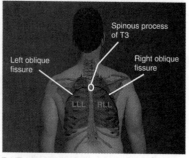

B. Posterior View

Figure 8-3 Lungs: RUL = Right Upper Lobe, RML = Right Middle Lobe, RLL = Right Lower Lobe, LUL = Left Upper Lobe, LLL = Left Lower Lobe.

8-3 depicts the location of the lobes, front and back.

Additional landmarks helpful in documenting assessment findings as well as in auscultation are illustrated in Figure 8-4. To find the right and left midclavicular line, locate the anterior clavicle and estimate midway. Draw an imaginary line vertically bisecting the ribs. Similarly, when locating the midaxillary line, draw an imaginary line between posterior and anterior axillary segments (Figure 8-4, C and D).

Health History Related to Respiratory Assessment

Symptom and disease-specific respiratory questions are asked to provide a starting point for inquiry prior to the respiratory

examination. Table 8-3 highlights priority data to ask the older adult.

Physical Examination of the Older Adult's Respiratory System

The four components of the physical examination (in this sequence)—inspection, palpation, percussion, and auscultation—pertain to the older adult. Be aware of how to manage the unique needs of some older adults, which require the nurse to adjust her or his approach to the respiratory examination. See Tables 8-4 through 8-10.

Flexibility and positional needs, cognitive and emotional deficits, and socially unacceptable behaviors associated with organic diseases affecting the brain all require special approaches in order to meet

✓ **NURSING CHECKLIST**

General Approach to Thorax and Lung Assessment

- Ensure that the examination room is well lit, quiet, and at a warm, comfortable temperature to prevent patient chilling and shivering.
- Instruct the patient to remove all street clothes from the waist up and to don an examination gown.
- Place the client in an upright sitting position on the examination table or rotate the supine patient from side to side to gain access to the thorax.
- Expose the entire area being assessed. For women, provide a drape to cover the breasts (if desired) when the posterior thorax is being assessed.
- When palpating, percussing, or auscultating the anterior thorax of female or obese patients, ask them to displace the breast tissue. Assessing directly over breast tissue does not yield accurate findings with regard to underlying structures.
- Visualize the underlying respiratory structures.
- Always compare the right and left sides of the anterior thorax and the posterior thorax to one another, as well as the right lateral thorax and the left lateral thorax.
- Use a systematic approach every time the assessment is performed. Proceed from the lung apices to the bases, right to left to lateral.

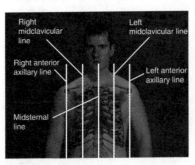

A. Anterior View

B. Posterior View

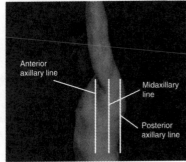

C. Right Lateral View

D. Left Lateral View

Figure 8-4   Imanginary Thoracic Lines

Table 8-3   Priority Respiratory Data to Elicit from the Older Adult

History of:
- Smoking
- Exercise, activity, and mobility levels
- Tuberculosis, asthma, chronic obstructive pulmonary disease (COPD), pneumonia, respiratory infections, lung cancer

Symptoms:
- Cough and nature of the cough
  - Phlegm production, color, odor, amount
  - Times of day

Dyspnea:
- Times of day
- Prompted by exertion, at rest, while asleep

Changes in respiratory rate:
- Below 12/minute or greater than 20/minute

Chest pain:
- Nature of the pain
- Not unique to bardiac problems in the older adult; may indicate respiratory problems such as pneumonia in the older adult

Adapted from Matteson, M., McConnell, M., & Linton, A. (1997). *Gerontological nursing: Concepts and practice,* Chapter 8. Philadelphia: W. B. Saunders.

the older adult's unique needs. Sometimes it is difficult to perform a respiratory examination on these individuals. The nurse may have to try at "better" times of day, or weigh the benefit-risk of the examination against clinical manifestations indicating treatment.

Of the four process components of the physical examination, percussion seems to be the least utilized, especially during a quick, episodic examination in the nursing home setting. *Listening* for adventitious sounds is probably the most utilized and *most critical skill* to master and holds the potential for reaping the most dramatic and lifesaving interventions, from both a medical and a nursing perspective. The breath sounds, as they pass through different densities of lung matter, from air to fluid to denser masses, imply degrees of functional capacity and diseases of the lungs relative to air exchange. In other words, lung *sounds* indicate efficiency in *travel* of gases exchange. Consider sound (auscultation) as a determinant of thickness and thus effectiveness of gas transfer; gases cannot travel effectively through dense matter. The presence of dense matter can be determined through percussion and somewhat through auscultation. If the nurse has "a good ear" for lung sounds, subtle respiratory and even cardiac changes are unveiled prior to major life-endangering events in the older adult.

Respiratory therapists are trained in implementing interventions related to asthma treatment, chronic obstructive pulmonary disease (COPD), and care of patients on ventilators. They work in collaboration with physicians, pulmonary specialists, nurses, anesthesiologists and physical therapists.

Table 8-4 Modifications to Make Based on the Challenging Needs of the Elite Older Adult	
1. Flexibility and positional needs	Some older adults may have limited movement and ability to sit up. Obtain assistance or examine in a side-to-side approach. If the older adult is very uncomfortable, delineate only what is important—adventitious breath sounds and abnormalities noted upon inspection and palpation.
2. Cognitive losses beyond normal age-related changes	If the older adult is unable to follow directions (i.e., take a deep breath, cough, etc.), normal inspiration/expiration will have to suffice. Again, differentiate between normal breath sounds and those which are adventitious.
3. Excessive anxiety or emotional dysfunction	Temporarily stop the exam. Spend time on another unrelated activity, preferably one that is soothing. perhaps a break is necessary. Sometimes incorporating the family member or significant other is helpful. However, there may not be one available.
4. Uninhibited behaviors	If the older adult does not have a sense of personal privacy, make sure you are in a room where the door can be closed. Also, provide quality examination gowns, which open in the front but which stay closed when necessary. Privacy and dignity have always been emphasized with all patients young and old. It becomes more of an issue when a person is unable to maintain his or her own privacy because of underlying cognitive diseases.

NURSING TIP

When teaching older adults about respiratory health, do not presume they are "too old to change." With internal motivation and a caring, unpressured environment, the older adult is permitted the *luxury* of deciding for himself or herself what is best. Promoting health in the older adult is all in the approach—the difference between preaching versus *teaching*.

Summary

Multiple skeletal and cellular age-related changes in the respiratory system of the older adult affect the process of air exchange within the lungs. Solid health history taking and physical examination are the basis for treatment and care. The "ideal" circumstances reuiring a mobile, flexable, and cognative older adult are usually models for the respiratory exam. However, the nurse must make significant alteration to accomodate the elite older adult.

Table 8-5   Steps of Respiratory Inspection and Abnormal Findings

Inspection:

Look at the anterior and posterior chest cavity. Are there any abnormalities including:

- Asymmetries
- Bulges
- Discolorations
- Bruises
- Excessive barrel chest beyond mild anterior-posterior chest widening (front to back is greater than side-to-side). In COPD ribs are pushed forward and outward giving a 1:1 ratio between AP and side-to-side diameter
- Depression or protrusion of the sternum
- Presence of visible veins and spider nevi (spider-like capillaries)
- Costal margin greater than 90 degrees, during exhalation, that is, with emphysema
- Ribs at 45 degree angle from sternum, horizontal protrusion, that is, with emphysema, cystic fibrosis, or hyperinflation of the bronchi
- Use of accessory muscles due to hypoxia caused from multiple pathologies such as pneumonia, pneumothorax, or COPD
- Respirations fewer than 12 or greater than 20 indicate respiratory distress
- Uneven respirations, that is, **Cheyne-Sokes** (deep and shallow breaths interspersed with periods of **apnea**)
- **Kussmaul's breathing** (deep and quick respirations) associated with diabetic ketoacidosis
- Labored respirations
- Excessive sighing
- Audible, noisy breathing heard greater than a few feet away may indicate COPD, pneumothorax, pneumonia, hypoxia, or nasal blockage/swelling
- Pursed-lip breathing seen in those with COPD to compensate for alveoli snapping shut too quickly
- Anything other than a small amount of light yellow to clear sputum

Summarized from Estes, M. E. Z. (1998). *Health assessment and physical examination.* Albany, NY: Delmar Publishers.

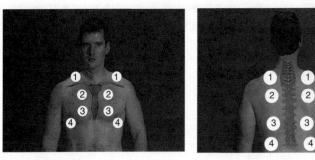

A. Anterior Thorax

B. Posterior Thorax

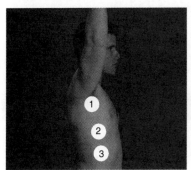

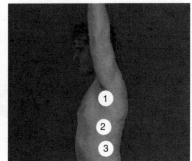

C. Right Lateral Thorax

D. Left Lateral Thorax

Figure 8-5   Pattern for Tactile Fremitus

Table 8-6   Steps of Respiratory Palpation and Abnormal Findings

Palpation:
Starting with anterior then to posterior chest, and under arms down midaxillary line, feel (using finger pads) for abnormalities, including:

- Clavicular or rib tenderness
- Tenderness at or around axilla and midaxillary line
- Presence of masses
- Crepitus, air that escapes into the subcutaneous tissue, feels like bubbles popping when palpating. May be due to air leakage from burst alveoli, chest trauma, or emphysema
- Uneven thoracic expansion when hands are butterflyed at the tenth rib, thumbs at the spine posteriorly, fingers spread in a "W"; same anteriorly may indicate scoliosis, pulmonary fibrosis, or any pulmonary disease whereby lungs are unable to expand
- Tactile fremitus (ask person to say "99" or "1-2-3") beyond a gentle vibration; palm of hand is placed at sites as shown in Figure 8-5 A through D.

Summarized from Estes, M. E. Z., (1998). *Health assessment and physical examination.* Albany, NY: Delmar Publishers.

Table 8-7 Summary of Percussion and Abnormalities

Percussion in older adults usually does not reap usable findings for the following reasons:

1. It is difficult to perform in some older adults because many are unable to assume required positions:

   - Upright
   - Arms folded
   - Head bent forward, significantly
   - Hands over head

2. Results are unreliable due to normal kyphosis and alveolar changes creating some hyperresonance (abnormal in adults).
3. Hyperresonance is also found in thin and less muscular adults, which then provides clinically ambiguous data.

Adapted from Matteson, M., McConnell, M., & Linton, A., (1997). *Gerontological nursing: Concepts and practice.* Philadelphia: W. B. Saunders.

Table 8-8 Normal and Adventitious Breath Sounds

I. Normal breath sounds:
  A. **Vesicular sounds:** soft, low, heard in lower portions of lungs
  B. **Bronchovesicular sounds:** moderate pitch and intensity, heard at middle portion of lungs
  C. **Bronchial sounds:** high-pitched, loud, heard over trachea

*Note: Each sound is *unique to its location,* that is, bronchial sounds should not be heard in the lower lobes. Also, large tubes (like the trachea) produce louder sounds: smaller structures produce softer, smoother sounds

II. Adventitious breath sounds
  A. **Crackles (rales):** fine and course
     - *Fine:* popping sounds, static-like, heard on inspiration
     - *Coarse:* moist, lower pitch, heard on inspiration
     - *Associated diseases:* congestive heart failure (CHF), pneumonia, COPD
  B. **Wheezes:** sonorous and sibilant
     - Sonorous (low-pitch, snoring, heard on expiration); associated with bronchitis, asthma, foreign body obstruction
     - Sibilant (high-pitch, musical, heard on expiration); associated with asthma, emphysema, bronchitis
  C. **Pleural friction rub:**
     - Sounds like a squeaky door, grating, heard at inspiration and expiration
     - Associated with pleurisy, tuberculosis, or inflamed pleural lining
  D. **Stridor:** crowing sound on inspiration
     - Associated with foreign body obstruction, large airway tumor

*Note: Crackles are discontinuous sounds whereas all others are continuous.

Adapted from Estes, M. E. Z., (1998). *Health assessment and physical examination.* Albany, NY: Delmar Publishers

---
Table 8-9   Steps of Auscultation and Abnormalities

I. While listening to each site in the sequence listed, compare breath sounds bilaterally:
- Ask the older adult to breathe through the mouth, inhaling and exhaling as the nurse moves to each site
- Monitor the older adult for hyperventilation and/or dizziness
- Auscultate, in this order: anterior, posterior, laterally

II. Listen for abnormalities:
- Adventitious breath sounds
- Vesicular, bronchial, or bronchovesicular sounds in places other than their normal location
- Decreased breath sounds (i.e., emphysema) or absence of breath sounds (atelectasis, tumor, pleural effusion)
- Voice sounds, determining densities of materials such as air or solids, are assessed if abnormalities are found during any part of the exam:
  - **Bronchophony**: stethoscope is placed at area of abnormality, patient says "99" or "1-2-3"
  - **Egophony**: same as above only patient says "ee"
  - Whispered pectoriloquy: same as above only patient whispers "99" or "1-2-3"

---
*"99"/"1-2-3" should sound muffled; if clear or very muffled, there is liquid or too much air in the lungs, respectively.

Table 8-10   Opportunities for Teaching Older Adults about Respiratory Health

---

When the older adult is receptive, offer information on:

1. Proper handwashing
2. Limiting exposure to large crowds during peak flu and cold seasons
3. Flu and pneumococcal pneumonia vaccines
4. Regular tuberculin testing
5. Smoking cessation tools
6. Avoiding environmental irritants, household chemical hazards, dust, pollen; having adequate inside ventilation
7. Exertion in excessively hot or cold weather
8. Smoke detector safety
9. Radon testing
10. Care of furnaces and heating devices, per manufacturer
11. Correct oxygen usage
12. balancing activity/exercise with respiratory capabilities

---

References

Estes, M. E. Z , (1998). *Health assessment & physical examination.* (pp. 365–401). Albany, NY: Delmar Publishers.

Matteson, M., McConnell, M., & Linton, A. (1997). Gerontological nursing: Concepts and practice. Philadelphia: W. B. Saunders.

Thomas, C. L. (1997). *Taber's cyclopedic medical dictionary* (18the ed.). Philadelphia: F. A. Davis Company.

9

Cardiovascular Assessment

Key Terms

aorta
atrioventricular (AV) node
atrium
capillary refill
cardiac cycle
coronary arteries
deep vein thrombosis (DVT)
heaves
Homan's sign
jugular vein pressure (JVP)
mitral valve
murmur
pericardial friction rub
precordium
pulmonic valve
pulsations
sinoatrial (SA) node
thrills
tricuspid valve
ventricle

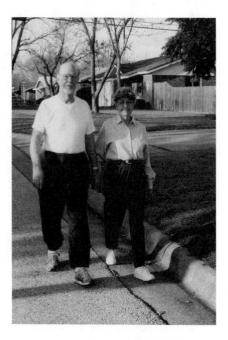

TIPS FROM THE EXPERTS

Falls in the older adult may be related to orthostatic hypotension, which is a drop in blood pressure and pulse when a person moves from a lying to a standing position. More than 10 mm Hg drop in systolic or diastolic pressure and an increase in heart rate of 20 beats or more indicate orthostatic hypotension. A lying, sitting, and standing blood pressure and pulse are taken to compare numbers related to symptoms of dizziness or weakness. Have the older adult lie down for 5 minutes; take the pulse and blood pressure; allow 2 or 3 minutes in between for sitting and standing results. Medications, fluid volume, and neurological problems are evaluated if orthostasis is discovered. Older adults should be instructed to sit a few minutes before standing.

The heart is associated with feelings of love, friendship, courage, and the human spirit. It is an amazing organ that has been crowned with literary and physiological praises. In spite of its size (approximately the size of a closed fist), it has the capacity to pump about 5 liters of blood within a minute. To varying degrees, the muscular ability of the heart, components of blood, and electrical conduction systems change as a person ages. In addition, peripheral vasculature, both arterial and venous in the lower extremities, narrows and loses resiliency as a person gets older.

Age-Related Changes in the Cardiovascular System of the Older Adult

Research on normal aging related to the cardiovascular (CV) system holds mixed results on what is *normal* versus changes related to *neglect* or *disuse*. There exists an extremely fine line between CV disease and the normal wear-and-tear of aging. It is hypothesized that CV age-related changes in older adults are somewhat reflective of a lifetime of health habits, combined with adaptive and compensatory mechanisms aimed at homeostasis. We do not fully understand these mechanisms. Findings on the effects of aerobic exercise, for example, indicate that many cardiovascular risk factors can be controlled. Research on exercise and on older athletes is most dramatic and impressive, supporting the implication that if humans commit to exercise, a low-fat diet, stress reduction, and overall maintenance of health, CV disease potentially might disappear, if not be drastically reduced. Tables 9-1 and 9-2 review age-related changes and CV risk factors, respectively.

Cardiac Cycle, Anatomical Landmarks, and Cardiac Conduction Systems

Systole and diastole comprise the **cardiac cycle.** Systole is the contraction phase of the heartbeat ("lub"), when blood empties from the ventricles; diastole is the relaxation phase ("dub"). Blood enters through the two atria. The tricuspid valve (separates right atria from right ventricle) and mitral valve (separates left atria from left ventricle) hold back blood until the atria are full, thus triggering an emptying into the ventricles. Blood leaves the heart by passing through the right ventricle, then through the pulmonic valve to be oxygenated by the lungs. Blood also pumps through the left ventricle and out to other body systems via the aortic valve.

The heart has its own network of arterial and venous circulation in the form of the coronary arteries and veins, the arteries of which encase the heart's outer surface. Figure 9-1 illustrates this system.

Electrical conduction initiates the rhythmic beat and steady contractions of the heart. The impulse begins in the **sinoatrial (SA) node.** The node tends to collect fatty deposits and thickens as people age, thus causing delays in conduction. From the SA node the impulse travels down to the **atrioventricular (AV) node** and bundle branch system, to the apex of the heart. Older adults are prone to cardiac arrhythmias, which are *not* part of normal, healthy aging. Figure 9-2 depicts each step of the electrical pathway of conduction.

Vasculature

For a review of the arterial and venous system and in preparation for finding arteries and veins during the CV exam, refer to Figures 9-3 and 9-4.

Cardiovascular History and Examination

The first portion of the CV assessment includes discussion with the older adult concerning health habits, previous history, and any symptoms. Table 9-3 lists priority data for the nurse to obtain.

The CV examination incorporates the skills of inspecting the **precordium,** palpating for abnormalities, and identifying abnormal heart sounds through auscultation. The second part includes assessing

Table 9-1   Summary of Cardiovascular Age-Related Changes in Older Adults

Decreases in:
- Release of calcium in the heart, prolonging contraction during systole
- Cardiac output at rest—*slight* decrease (mixed research results)
- Baroreceptor sensitivity (baroreceptor cells help regulate blood pressure), possibly readjusted as a result of a thicker, stiffer aorta and overall aging of nerve cells
- Left ventricular filling in diastole
- Hematocrit, hemoglobin, lymphocytes are slightly decreased

Increases in:
- Calcification and stiffening of the heart valves (aortic and mitral)
- Thickness in left ventricle wall, small increase
- Increase in atria (slight) with late diastolic filling to compensate for slowing of left ventricular filling; may result in S4 sound (atrial gallop)
- Fibrous tissue in the heart
- Amyloid tissue in the heart (debatable whether this is part of normal aging)
- Systolic and diastolic murmurs from ineffective valve closure
- Vessel rigidity in aorta
- Peripheral vascular resistance (mixed research findings; same versus increases)
- Blood pressure, slight increase
- Blood coagulation
- Fatty cells in the sinoatrial (SA) node, replacing pacer cells
- Electrocardiographic abnormalities
  - PR and QT intervals increase
  - Propensity for arrythmias

Summarized from Abrams, W., Beers, M., & Berkow, R. (Eds.). (1995). *The Merck manual of geriatrics* (2nd ed.) Rahway, NJ: Merck Research Laboratories; and Matteson, M., McConnell, M., & Linton, A. (1997). *Gerontological nursing: Concepts and practice*, (Chapter 7). Philadelphia: W. B. Saunders.

for **jugular vein pressure (JVP)** and precise palpation of pulses.

Precordium Assessment

As in any examination and assessment of body systems, a step-by-step approach is preferable, unless behavioral, emergency, or other situations pose barriers. The precordium is inspected and auscultated using the landmarks indicated in Figure 9-5.

Although the landmarks do not represent the locations of the valves, it is where they are most audible.

Inspection

In an adequately lit room, ask the older adult to lie flat (supine). Locate each of five landmarks in Figure 9-6, and lightly palpate, then observe each for **pulsations (visible pulsing movement).** Pulsations in any of the five areas are abnormal, with the exception of the mitral area. All of the precordium should remain "still" except for the mitral area if the apex of the heart is close to the surface. Pulsations may indicate the following abnormalities:

Table 9-2   Review of Cardiovascular Risk Factors

High-risk profile:
- Inactivity, sedentary lifestyle
- Smoker
- Male, or female post-menopausal, or female smoker on birth control pills
- African American
- Obese
- High blood pressure
- Diabetes
- Under stress
- Hyperlipidemia
- Family history of heart disease

*Note that all except family history, gender, and race can be controlled.

🜂 NURSING ALERT

Warning Signs of Imminent Cardiovascular Problems

- Change in color of the lips, face, or nails
- Chest pain
- Extreme diaphoresis
- Dizziness
- Dyspnea
- Edema
- Exremity pain
- Fatigue
- Feelings of doom
- Numbness in the extremities
- Pain that limits self-care
- Palpitations
- Syncope
- Tingling in the extremities

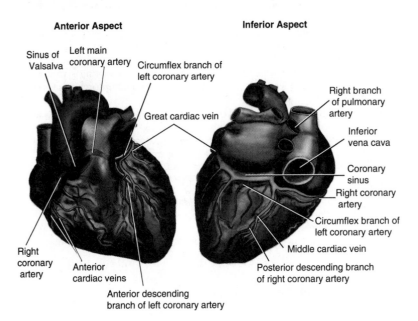

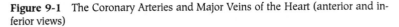

Figure 9-1   The Coronary Arteries and Major Veins of the Heart (anterior and inferior views)

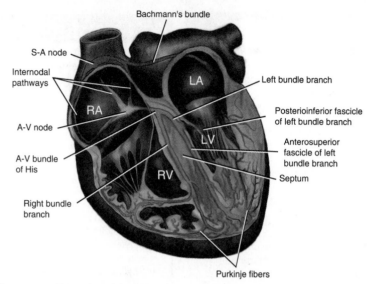

Figure 9-2   Excitation of the Heart

Table 9-3   Priority Cardiovascular Data to Obtain from the Older Adult

Cardiac history of:
- Dizziness, lightheadedness, syncope, edema (look for inability to get shoes on due to swelling)
- Hypertension (HTN)
- Previous myocardial infarction (MI) and type of presenting symptoms (note that the older adult presents atypically: no symptoms to classic symptoms)
- Coronary artery disease (CAD), angina, previous cerebral vascular accident (CVA) or transient ischemic attack (TIA)
- Mitral stenosis, mitral valve replacement, murmurs (up to 60 percent of older adults have murmurs)
- Sick sinus syndrome, pacer insertion (permanent or temporary)

History of:
- Current medications and laboratory tests including;
  - Triglycerides
  - Cholesterol
  - HDL/LDL ratio (high-density lipoprotein/low-density lipoprotein)
- Obesity
- Inactivity
- Stress
- Alcohol (ETOH) and tobacco usage

Pulmonary symptoms:
- Dyspnea, and when it occurs
- Orthopnea; use of multiple pillows while sleeping
- Shortness of breath and, when it occurs, wheezing

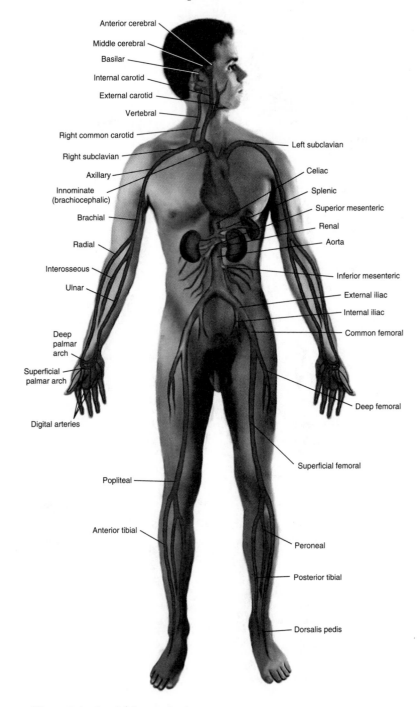

Figure 9-3   Arterial System Anatomy

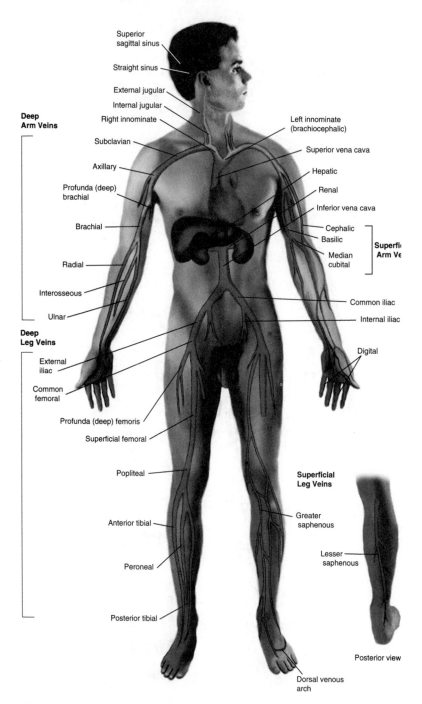

Figure 9-4   Venous System Anatomy

- Aortic aneurysm
- Ventricular aneurysm
- Right ventricular enlargement
- Mitral regurgitation

It is not uncommon to observe some cardiac pulsations and abnormalities, especially in the elite older adult or nursing home resident. In these cases, disease processes have progressed with surgical interventions yielding minimal benefit to quality of life.

Palpation

Using the same five landmarks (see Figure 9-5) ("A-P-E-T-M" mnemonic; Figure 9-6), palpate for three sensations: **pulsations, thrills** (a "motor-like" vibration palpated with the palm of the hand), and **heaves** (a lift in the area of palpation; indicates the heart is working very hard to pump blood). Again, the older adult is in a supine position. There should be no palpable pulsations, thrills, or heaves unless disease is present; pulsation may be palpated in the mitral area at the apex of the heart but no thrill or heave should be felt. If the apical pulse cannot be felt, ask the older adult to roll onto his or her left side. This moves the heart closer to the surface

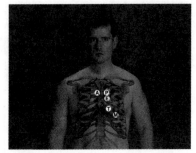

Figure 9-5   Auscultation Landmarks

of the chest, making palpation easier. Commonly found problems may include:

- Aortic stenosis/regurgitation, felt as a thrill
- Pulmonic stenosis/regurgitation, felt as a thrill
- Enlarged right ventricle or left ventricular aneurysm, felt as a heave
- Mitral stenosis/regurgitation, felt as a thrill

Auscultation

Using the same five cardiac landmarks, listen to the heart with either the bell or diaphragm of the stethoscope while the

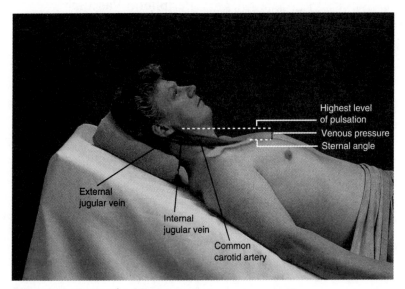

Highest level
of pulsation

Venous pressure

Sternal angle

External
jugular vein

Internal
jugular vein

Common
carotid artery

Figure 9-6   Position for JVP Measurement

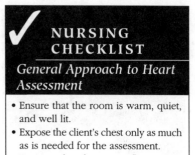

✓ **NURSING CHECKLIST**

General Approach to Heart Assessment

• Ensure that the room is warm, quiet, and well lit.
• Expose the client's chest only as much as is needed for the assessment.
• Position the client in a flat, supine position.
• Stand to the client's right side. In order to accentuate shadows, the light should come from the opposite side of where you are standing.

older adult is in a sitting position, or, if necessary, a supine position. Auscultation is a sophisticated skill. Listen for each heart sound separately. Take one or 2 minutes, *at least,* to auscultate. Start with either the mitral area and work upward, or the aorta area and move downward. The following section will cover the basics of the four "S" sounds, murmurs, and pericardial friction rub.

The Four "S" Sounds

S1 and S2 represent the normal heart sounds of systole and diastole—the "lub-dub." Regardless of age, "lub-dub" indicates normal heart functioning. Generally, S3 and S4 are considered abnormal heart sounds in older adults indicative of cardiac and fluid overload (S3/mimics the word, "Kentucky"), as in congestive heart failure, or aortic stenosis and ventricular failure (S4/gallop/mimics the word, "Tennessee"), as in cardiomyopathy or myocardial infarction. Table 9-4 summarizes where the four heart sounds, murmurs, and pericardial friction rub are best heard. For more information on auscultation, the nurse clinical specialist may want to refer to heart sound tapes and a separate cardiac assessment reference text.

Murmurs

Murmurs are caused by blockage, obstruction, or abnormal backward/front-

ward blood flow in the heart. Murmurs do not necessarily correspond with the heart beat, but sound like "swishing." They are best heard in the four areas of the **valves: aortic, pulmonic, tricuspid,** and **mitral areas.** Use the diaphragm of the stethoscope for the aortic and pulmonic areas and the bell of the stethoscope for the mitral and tricuspid areas. Murmurs, which may be considered normal in children, are an abnormal finding in older adults. Describe murmurs using the seven characteristics in Table 9-5.

Pericardial Friction Rub

For auscultation for the presence of a **pericardial friction rub,** have the older adult sit up, leaning forward. The sound of a friction rub is similar to a high-pitched, grating noise. Listen at the third to fifth intercostal space on the sternum, then move down in steps as a pathway motion to the mitral area, which tracks the lining of the pericardium. Pericarditis or kidney failure may be associated with the presence of a pericardial friction rub. Unlike a *pleural* friction rub, the *pericardial* friction rub is high-pitched and remains constant with respirations.

Peripheral Vascular Assessment

Peripheral vascular assessment in the older adult includes palpation and auscultation of pulses (arterial) and inspection of jugular venous pressure.

Assessment of Pulses

Left ventricular function is reflected in arterial pulse assessment. Using the index and middle finger, palpate these pulses:

• Temporal carotid
• Brachial
• Radial
• Femoral
• Popliteal
• Posterior tibial
• Dorsalis pedis

Refer to Figure 4-1 and Table 4-1.

sTable 9-4	Remembering the 'What' and 'Where' of Heart Sounds			
	Aortic Area	Pulmonic Area	Tricuspid Area	Mitral Area
S2 (diastole/"dub")	X	X		
S1 (systole/"lub")			X (softer)	X (louder)
S3 (abnormal) Early diastolic filing sound: "Kentucky" S1-S2-S3			X	X
S4 (abnormal) Late diastolic filling sound: "Tennessee" S4-S1-S2			X Use bell of stethoscope	X Use bell of stethoscope
Murmurs (swishing sound)	X Use diaphragm of stethoscope	X Use diaphragm of stethoscope	X Use bell and diaphragm of stethoscope	X Use bell and diaphragm of stethoscope
Pericardial friction rub: Grating sound		X	X	X

Rate, rhythm, amplitude, and *symmetry* are noted. Rate is beats per minute. Rhythm is regularity versus irregularity. Symmetry denotes equal rates bilaterally. Amplitude is the strength or pressure felt from the pulse. A scale is sometimes used to rate amplitude (see Table 9-7).

Bruits (blowing sounds connoting obstruction) should be auscultated using the bell of the stethoscope; listen to the temporal, carotid, and femoral arteries. No sounds should be heard in these arteries.

It is important to assess extremities in the older adult to determine whether tissues farthest from the heart are being perfused. Examine nailbeds for **capillary refill** by pressing down on the nail for a few seconds. Then release pressure. The nailbed should go from blanched to pink within 2 to 3 seconds. In addition, test for **Homan's sign** by quickly pulling back (dorsiflexing) the older adult's foot while she or he is in a supine position. Pain indicates a positive Homan's sign. Although current research shows that a positive Homan's sign is not a reliable indicator of

Table 9-5	The Seven Characteristics of Murmurs

- Location: Where is the murmur best heard?
- Radiation: Where does the sound radiate to? Chest wall? Axilla?
- Timing: Is it a systolic murmur (occurs with the pulse)? Diastolic murmur (does not occur with the pulse)?
- Intensity: What is the degree of loudness? Grades I–VI (see Table 9-6)
- Quality: Is the sound harsh, rumbling, blowing, or musical?
- Pitch: Is the pitch of the sound high, medium, or low?
- Configuration: What is the pattern of the sound? Loud to soft (decrescendo) or soft to loud (crescendo)?

Adapted from Estes, M. E. Z., (1998). *Health assessment and physical examination.* (434–435) Albany: Delmar Publishers.

Table 9-6 Grading Heart Murmurs	
Grade	Characteristics
I	Very faint; heard only after a period of concentration
II	Faint; heard immediately
III	Moderate intensity
IV	Loud; may be associated with a thrill
V	Loud; stethoscope must remain in contact with the chest wall in order to hear; thrill palpable
VI	Very loud; heard with stethoscope off chest wall; thrill palpable

Table 9-7   Scales for Measuring Pulse Volume

3-POINT SCALE

Scale	Description of Pulse
0	Absent
1+	Thready/weak
2+	Normal
3+	Bounding

4-POINT SCALE

Scale	Description of Pulse
0	Absent
1+	Thready/weak
2+	Normal
3+	Increased
4+	Bounding

deep vein thrombosis (DVT), clinicians may or may not incorporate it into their assessment. Opinion is mixed.

Continue to inspect the extremities for ulcerations, color, and edema. Venous ulcerations are usually found on ankles and shins whereas arterial ulcers are located at the far extremities (tips of fingers and toes). Feet are often a forgotten part of the body. If ulceration is present, a person may intentionally bandage and cover the ulcer. It is critical that the nurse inspects the feet carefully. Feet help ensure mobil-

---

NURSING TIP

Pericardial Friction Rub Versus Pleural Friction Rub

- A pericardial friction rub produces a *high*-pitched, multiphasic, scratchy (may be leathery or grating) sound that *does not* change with respiration. It is a sign of pericardial inflammation.
- A pleural friction rub produces a *low*-pitched, coarse, grating sound that *does* change with respiration. When the patient holds his or her breath, the sound disappears. The patient may also complain of pain upon breathing. It is a sign of visceral and parietal pleurae inflammation.

---

ity; loss of a foot for an older adult can mean loss of mobility and reduced functional status. Moreover, independence and self-concept are threatened.

Edema is assessed by pressing with the index finger on the legs, hands, and sacrum. If indentation is noted after releasing the pressure, pitting edema is present. Pitting edema is described as 0–+1 (mild, 1/4 inch)–+2 (moderate, 1/2 inch)–+3 (severe, 1 inch)–+4 (severe, greater than 1 inch pitting). No or very mild edema is a normal finding in older adults.

Assessing Jugular Vein Pressure

Measuring jugular vein pressure (JVP) helps the nurse add to the clinical picture relative to cardiac efficiency, especially right ventricular function, vein obstruction, and/or increased blood volume. Figure 9-6 depicts the position whereby JVP can be best observed and measured.

Visually observe for pulsations, bilaterally. In centimeters, measure the distance in *height* between the top of the sternal angle and the highest point where the jugular vein is noted. Add 5 centimeters to your measurement because the location of the right atrium is about 5 centimeters under the sternal angle. A measurement greater than 9 centimeters is considered abnormal.

In addition to assessing JVP, the nurse may also want to test for hepatojugular reflux, indicative of right ventricular failure. While the older adult is at a 30 degree angle, apply deep palpation on the right upper quadrant of the abdomen for about a minute. Release. Observe the neck for increased pulsation/jugular vein pressure.

Health Teaching

Remember that older adults are not "too old" to learn positive health habits. Furthermore, they are not "too old" to change, if internally and externally motivated to do so. Controlling cardiac risk factors and supporting cardiovascular interventions should not be abandoned just because someone is 90 years old.

References

Abrams, W., Beers, M., & Berkow, R. (Eds.). (1995). *The Merck manual of geriatrics* (2nd ed.). Rahway, NJ: Merck Research Laboratories.

Cauthorne-Burnette, T. & Estes, M. E. Z., (1998). *Clinical companion for health assessment and physical examination.* Albany, NY: Delmar Publishers.

Estes, M. E. Z., (1998). *Health assessment and physical examination* (Chapter 15). Albany, NY: Delmar Publishers.

Matteson, M., McConnell, M., & Linton, A. (1997). *Gerontological nursing concepts and practice.* Chapter 7. Philadelphia: W. B. Saunders.

10

Breast and Nodes Assessment

Key Terms

areola
breast self-examination (BSE)
central axillary nodes
Cooper's ligaments
gynecomastia
infraclavicular nodes
lateral nodes
lymph nodes
mastectomy
papilloma
pectoral nodes
subscapular nodes
supraclavicular nodes
tail of Spence

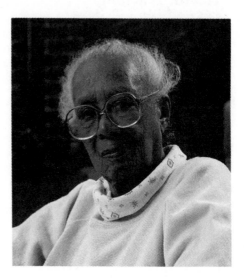

Introduction

The focus of Chapter 10 is on supporting breast health in women and men. Breast tissue, surrounding muscles and lymph nodes are discussed. Breast self-examination is described as an essential skill for both older women and older men to prevent breast cancer and promote self-care.

Breast tissue

The breasts and mammary glands of a woman are located on the anterior chest and extend laterally to the axilla and vertically from the second to sixth rib. The quadrants of the breast, supporting musculature, and glandular tissue are shown in Figures 10-1, 10-2, and 10-3.

The male breast is less developed than the female breast. The nipple is smaller but the **areola** is larger. Enlarged breast tissue or **gynecomastia,** may be seen in adolescent and older males. Body image in older adult males is affected by gynecomastia. Likewise, changes in the breast tissue and supportive structure in females contributes to alteration in body image. Table 10-1 lists age-related changes

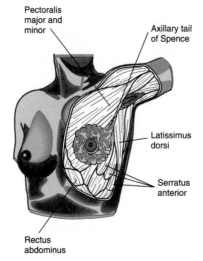

Figure 10-2   Muscles Supporting the Breast

in breast and lymph nodes unique to older women.

Regional Lymph Nodes

The lymph nodes drain toxins and other waste materials from the surrounding tissue. Relative to the breasts, the lymphatic

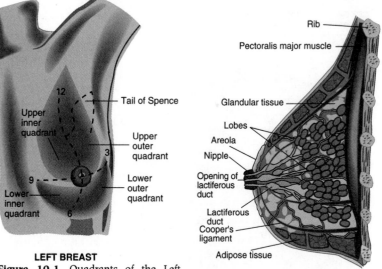

LEFT BREAST
Figure 10-1   Quadrants of the Left Breast

Figure 10-3   Glandular Tissue

Table 10-1   Normal Age-Related Changes in Breast Tissue of Women

- Atrophy of mammary tissue
- Increase in adipose tissue
- Slight decrease in breast size
- Some elongation and flattening of breast
- Some flattening of the nipple

network is located in four main areas: axillary, **pectoral, subscapular,** and **lateral,** as shown in Figure 10-4.

Inspection of the Breast

Many older men and women maintain a high degree of modesty, and may be embarrassed about their bodies. Religious beliefs, social mores, and overall patterns of behavior associated with body image, aging, and self-esteem influence an older adult's comfort with breast examination (self or by a nurse). Respect the older adult's value system and dignity by maintaining the highest level of privacy. Provide a robe or cover shirt, removing it only while performing the examination. During the examination, explain actions. This serves a dual purpose: to allay the client's nervousness or embarrassment and to teach the client the method of examination.

While facing the seated client with the client's arms relaxed at sides, inspect the breasts for symmetry, size, skin color, areolar and nipple color, edema, vascularity lesions or unusual bulges/masses, scarring, and drainage from the nipples. Slight asymmetry is normal; *perfectly* symmetrical breasts are an unusual finding. Ask the client to raise arms over head, and inspect. The axillae and contour of the breasts are viewed more clearly with arms raised. Both positions of inspection are depicted in Figures 10-5 and 10-6.

If the older adult is unable to raise arms over head, try to gently raise arms without forcing the movement. Ask the client to press hands into hips, which accentuates tissue masses and possible retraction surrounding the musculature. Refer to Figure 10-7.

The final position in inspection of breasts is the forward position. The breasts will hang freely from the chest wall, again emphasizing subtle yet visible masses or dimpling. See Figure 10-8.

Palpation of the Breast and Nodes

There are four areas of palpation:

- **supraclavicular** and **infraclavicular** lymph nodes
- breasts, with arms at side, then arms over head
- axillary lymph nodes
- breasts, with client in supine position

The regional lymph nodes are shown in Figure 10-4.

Palpation of the supraclavicular and infraclavicular nodes are performed with the client in a seated position as shown in Figures 10-9 and 10-10, respectively.

Upon palpation, findings of greater than approximately 1 centimeter nodes may indicate an abnormality such as metastases or lymphoma. Pain when palpating may indicate an infectious process or carcinoma in an older adult.

Palpation of the breasts in a sitting po-

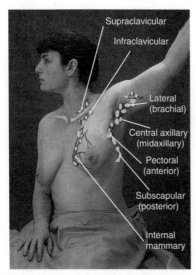

Supraclavicular
Infraclavicular
Lateral (brachial)
Central axillary (midaxillary)
Pectoral (anterior)
Subscapular (posterior)
Internal mammary

Figure 10-4   Regional Lymphatics

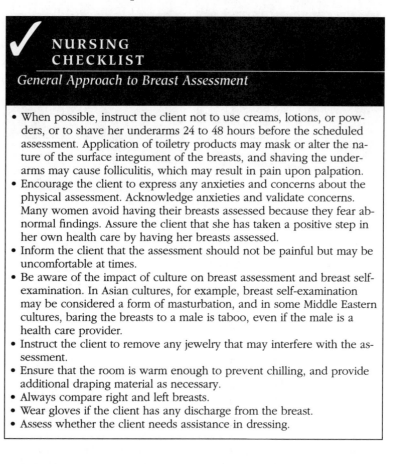

✓ **NURSING CHECKLIST**

General Approach to Breast Assessment

- When possible, instruct the client not to use creams, lotions, or powders, or to shave her underarms 24 to 48 hours before the scheduled assessment. Application of toiletry products may mask or alter the nature of the surface integument of the breasts, and shaving the underarms may cause folliculitis, which may result in pain upon palpation.
- Encourage the client to express any anxieties and concerns about the physical assessment. Acknowledge anxieties and validate concerns. Many women avoid having their breasts assessed because they fear abnormal findings. Assure the client that she has taken a positive step in her own health care by having her breasts assessed.
- Inform the client that the assessment should not be painful but may be uncomfortable at times.
- Be aware of the impact of culture on breast assessment and breast self-examination. In Asian cultures, for example, breast self-examination may be considered a form of masturbation, and in some Middle Eastern cultures, baring the breasts to a male is taboo, even if the male is a health care provider.
- Instruct the client to remove any jewelry that may interfere with the assessment.
- Ensure that the room is warm enough to prevent chilling, and provide additional draping material as necessary.
- Always compare right and left breasts.
- Wear gloves if the client has any discharge from the breast.
- Assess whether the client needs assistance in dressing.

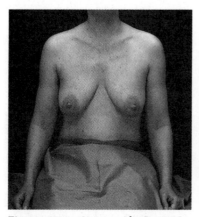

Figure 10-5 Arms-at-side Breast Inspection

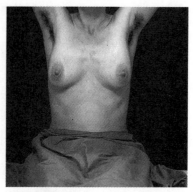

Figure 10-6 Arms-overhead Breast Inspection

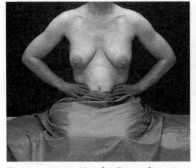

Figure 10-7 Hands Pressed against Hips

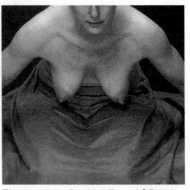

Figure 10-8 Leaning Forward Position

sition and with arms raised is an important detail of the exam. This is illustrated in Figure 10-11.

The outer quadrant of the breast is palpated, proceeding inward toward the sternal border while the breast is supported with the opposite hand. Repeat the assessment with the arms raised. Again, it must be noted that some older adults may be uncomfortable with such an intimate examination. Limited range of motion may prohibit raising the arms. Similarly, it may not be possible to proceed with the examination on older adults with moderate to more pronounced degrees of dementia. Judgment, sensitivity, and encouragement are important nursing interventions during the examination.

Axillary lymph nodes are examined next by beginning palpation at the apex of

the axilla, working downward through the four groups of axillary nodes:

- **posterior (subscapular)**
- **central (midaxillary)**
- **anterior (pectoral)**
- **lateral (brachial)**

Figure 10-12 depicts palpation of the axillary nodes.

The final step in palpation proceeds with the older adult in a supine position. As breast tissue gently falls to the sides, abnormalities become more visible. Each breast is palpated either concentrically or in wedge segments. The mammary tissues are gently compressed against the chest wall. A reduction in fat and subcutaneous tissue contributes to more obvious observance and palpation of masses in the older

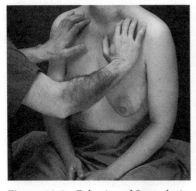

Figure 10-9 Palpation of Supraclavicular Nodes

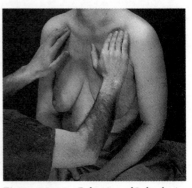

Figure 10-10 Palpation of Infraclavicular Nodes

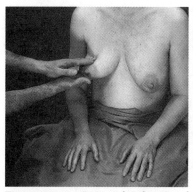

Figure 10-11 Bimanual Palpation of the Breasts while Patient is Sitting

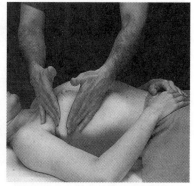

A. Palpation of the Glandular Area

adult. Figures 10-13A, B, and C indicate palpation of the glandular tissue, areola, and nipple in the supine position. A hardening and thickening of the nipple along with discharge may indicate a tumor or **papilloma.** Some medications, including diuretics, digitalis, steroids, tricyclics, oral contraceptives, chlorpromazine, and alpha-methlydopa, may precipitate nipple discharge. Note that the nurse is wearing gloves as a precaution because of possible drainage from the nipple.

Abnormal findings are summarized in Table 10-2.

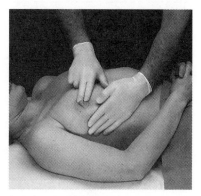

B. Palpation of the Areola

Breast Self-Examination and Education

Although breast self-examination (BSE) teaching efforts are not aimed at the older

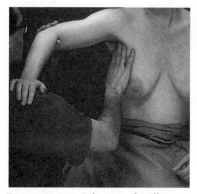

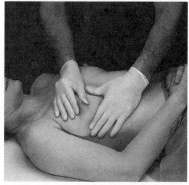

C. Compression of the Nipple while Patient is Supine

Figure 10-12 Palpation of Axillary Nodes '

Figure 10-13 Palpation of the Breast while Client is Supine

Table 10-2   Abnormal Inspection and Palpation, Breast and Node Findings in an Older Woman

- Reddened areas (breast, nipple, axillae)
- Striae unilaterally over breast or axilla
  —darker color in dark-skinned-persons
  —lighter color in light-skinned persons
- Unilateral vascularity
- Edema and thickening of tissue
  —orange rind appearance *(peau d'orange)*
- Asymmetrical nipple direction
- Change in shape of nipple, erosion of nipple
- Dimpling or retraction of breast
- Lesions/masses
- Palpable nodes > 1 centimeter in diameter

Adapted from Estes, M. E. Z., (1998). *Health assessment and physical examination.* Albany, NY: Delmar Publishers.

NURSING TIP

The Client with a Known Breast Mass

If the client has a known mass or irregularity in one breast, begin palpation on the unaffected breast. The unaffected breast should indicate the patient's normal physiological state.

⚘ NURSING ALERT

Risk Factors for Breast Cancer

- Over 50 years of age; risk increases with age
- Personal history of breast cancer
- Mother, grandmother, or sister with breast cancer
- Menarche at an early age, menopause at an advanced age
- High-fat diet
- Obesity
- Alcohol intake of greater than three servings per day
- American or European descent
- Urban dweller
- Estrogen therapy
- Nulliparous
- First birth after age 30
- Higher education and socioeconomic status

adult population, it is paramount to teach this brief and easy technique to clients who are receptive, capable, interested, and motivated to take responsibility for their body and their health. As individuals age, their likelihood of encountering cancer increases. Breast cancer is treatable in older adults. It is also preventable. Both men and women should be taught the technique (Hoskins & Haber, 2000). Approximately one percent of men will encounter breast cancer.

The nurse is likely to encounter clients who have had mastectomies. There are three types: **simple mastectomy** (breast is removed), **modified radical procedure** (breast and lymphs removed), and **subcutaneous mastectomy** (skin and nipple are intact with removal of underlying tissue and lymphs). BSE is encouraged in individuals who have experienced a mastectomy to help determine whether new masses have recurred. The Nursing Alert avove and Nursing Tip following describe risk factors and BSE to help strategize teaching plans for older adults.

References

Cauthorne-Burnette, T., & Estes, M. E. Z., (1998). *Clinical companion for health assessment and physical examination.* Albany, NY: Delmar Publishers.

Estes, M. E. Z., (1998). *Health assessment and physical examination.* Albany, NY: Delmar Publishers.

Hoskins, C. N., & Haber, J. (2000). Adjusting to breast cancer. *AJN, 100*(4), 26–32.

NURSING TIP

Breast Self-Examination (BSE)

Teaching BSE can be quick and simple.

1. Breast self-examination should be performed once a month, or on any given fixed date. Encourage her to put the BSE on her calendar and to include her significant other in the process.
2. *B (bed):* Show the client how to use the palmar surfaces of her fingers to palpate her breast while lying supine in bed. She should start by placing her right arm over her head and palpating her right breast with her left hand, moving in concentric circles from the periphery inward and including the periphery, tail of Spence, and areola. Finally, instruct her to squeeze the nipple to check for discharge. Using the reverse procedure, she should examine the other breast.
3. *S (standing):* Instruct the client to repeat the above palpation method while standing.
4. *E (examination in front of a mirror):* The client should stand in front of a mirror, first with her arms at her sides, then with her arms raised over her head, and finally with her hands pressed into her hips. She should examine her breasts for symmetry, retraction, dimpling, inverted nipples, and nipple deviation.

11

Musculoskeletal and Functional Assessment

Key Terms

abduction
activities of daily living (ADLs)
adduction
ankylosis
carpal tunnel syndrome
cortical bone
crepitus
degenerative joint disease (DJD)
external rotation
forward flexion
functional status
Heberden's nodes
hyperextension
instrumental activities of daily living
    (IADLs)
internal rotation
kyphosis
occupational therapist
olecranon processes
osteoarthritis
osteoporosis
Paget's disease
physical therapist
range of motion (ROM)
scoliosis
spinal processes
subluxation
Thomas test
trabecular bone

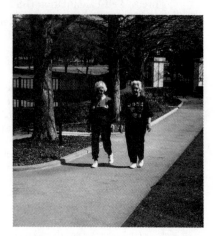

TIPS FROM THE EXPERTS

When performing a musculoskeletal examination, explain every step of the procedure *in advance*. Palpating and touching the body from behind or even in front of a person invades personal space and may frighten some individuals if they do not know what to expect. Stop if the person is experiencing pain.

The muscles and bones comprise the frame of the body, facilitating movement and expression. The 206 bones and over 600 muscles protect and hold the soft organs in place in conjunction with the skin. Figures 11-1 and 11-2 (A and B) show the anatomical structures of bones and muscles.

Age-Related Changes

Age-related changes in bones and muscles influence an older person's **functional status.** The effect on mobility, flexibility, and **range of motion (ROM)** directly pace the fun-filled activities, which the older person is able to participate in and enjoy. Individuals who continue to maintain an active lifestyle from their middle years are likely to enjoy optimum functional status throughout their later years. Do not expect someone who never golfed to start doing so, unless she or he is uniquely motivated. Therefore, it is paramount that younger individuals develop active lifestyles that are likely to enhance and influence the later years. Table 11-1 summarizes age-related muscle and bone changes.

Pertinent Health History Data

Table 11-2 identifies important elements when obtaining a health history.

Table 11-3 lists the most commonly used terms to describe joint movement.

Musculoskeletal Assessment

There are three dimensions of musculoskeletal assessment: general, specific, and functional.

General musculoskeletal assessment comprises inspection of overall appearance, posture, gait and mobility, and joint function. Specific assessment requires testing joints and muscles. Functional assessment requires collecting data about activities of daily living.

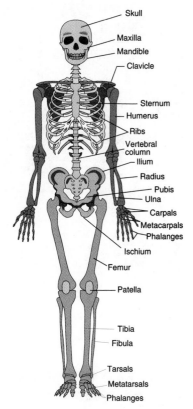

Figure 11-1 Adult skeleton: Anterior view

General Musculoskeletal Assessment

Obtain the height and weight of the older person. Guessing whether a person is overweight or underweight is not a reliable method of assessment. If the person is in a wheelchair and unable to stand, determine the weight of the wheelchair and subtract it from the total weight. Special scales are made for clients in a wheelchair or bed. Make a notation of clothing worn while weighing the person.

Note whether the person is able to bear weight while standing, with or without assistance. In addition, identify posture or any structural abnormalities, such as **kyphosis,** upon inspection. Posture is

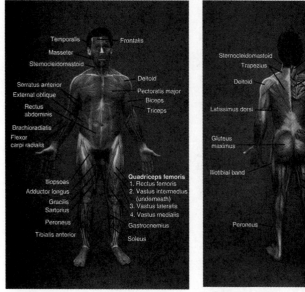
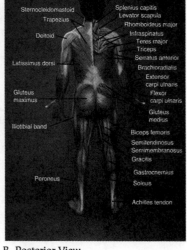

A. Anterior View

B. Posterior View

Figure 11-2   Muscles of the Body

Table 11-1   Summary of Age-Related Musculoskeletal Changes

Decreases in:
- Height (range of 2 to 4 inches from spinal column)
- **Trabecular** and **cortical bone,** especially in vertebrae, wrist, and hip
- Overall movement (slows)
- Strength (varies)
    - ↓Type II muscle fibers and isometric strength
    - ↓high-speed performance
- ↓reflexes
- ↓lean body mass
- ↓joint capsule (at elbows, knees, and wrists)

Increases in:
- cartilage: ears and nose broadens
- calcium loss from bones
- flexion of joints (**ankylosis:** stiffening of ligaments and joints)
- pelvis widens (but shoulders narrow)
- muscular wasting
- subcutaneous fat, especially at hips and abdomen
- bony prominences (more notable)
- resting tremors
- no change in long bones

Adapted from Matteson, M., McConnell, E. S., & Linton, A. D. (1997). *Gerontological nursing: Concepts and practice.* Philadelphia: W. B. Saunders.

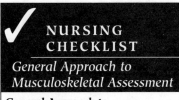

NURSING CHECKLIST

General Approach to Musculoskeletal Assessment

General Approach to Musculoskeletal Assessment

- Assist the client into a position of comfort.
- Be clear in your instructions to the client if you are asking her or him to perform a certain body movement or to assume a certain position. Demonstrate the desired movement if necessary.
- Notify the client before touching or manipulating a painful body part.
- Inspection, palpation, ROM, and muscle testing are performed on the major skeletal muscles and joints of the body in a cephalocaudal, proximal-to-distal manner. Always compare paired muscles and joints.
- Examine nonaffected body parts before affected body parts.
- Avoid unnecessary or excessive manipulation of a painful body part. If the client complains of pain, stop the aggravating motion.
- Some musculoskeletal disorders affect the client more during certain times of the day. Arrange for the follow-up appointment to be during the client's time of optimal function.

Table 11-2 Summary of Health History Data Related to Musculoskeletal Status

Note medical history of the following:
- **Osteoporosis** or **osteoarthritis**
- Rheumatoid arthritis
- **Paget's disease**
- Chronic low back pain
- Chronic muscle spasms or cramps
- **Scoliosis** or **kyphoscoliosis**
- Polymyalgia
- Gout
- **Carpal tunnel syndrome**
- Multiple sclerosis, amotrophic lateral sclerosis (ALS)

Surgical history of:
- Joint replacement
- Open reduction and internal fixation (ORIF)
- Laminectomy, spinal fusion
- Torn rotator cuff repair
- Debridement
- Limb/digit amputation or reattachment

Other:
- Fractures, tendon tears, spinal cord injury
- Back injury
- Cartilage damage
- Need for brace or splint

best examined by standing in front of the client and asking him or her to stand and sit while noting position of head, torso, and limbs. Arms should hang evenly; head, shoulders, hips, knees, and toes should point forward, symmetrically. Many older adults have a wide base of support because of widening of the pelvis, which may affect balance and gait.

Signs of pain (such as grimacing, shifting of position) are essential to note. Some older individuals accept pain as a normal part of aging and thus do not verbalize their discomfort. Ask the older person if she/he is in pain.

Asking the older person to walk to a landmark in the room, turn around, and walk back tests gait and mobility. The nurse may also instruct the person to walk on toes and heels, if appropriate. Gait should appear smooth, using heel-toe action. Arms should swing easily. The client should not bump into surrounding furniture but should move around it, sensing spatial boundaries. Joint diseases, Parkinson's, and Alzheimer's disease influence gait patterns. Refer to Table 11-4 for examples of abnormal gait patterns.

Although many older individuals manifest muscle atrophy, contour should be evident. Exercise and lifestyle affect muscle size and shape. Immobility, sedentary

Table 11-3   Descriptive Terms for Joint Range of Motion

Term	Description	Change in Joint Angle
Flexion	Bending of a joint so that the articulating bones on either side of the joints are moved closer together	Decreased
Extension	Bending the joint so that the articulating bones on either side of the joint are moved farther apart	Increased
Hyperextension	Extension beyond the neutral position	Increased beyond the angle of extension
Adduction	Moving the extremity medially and toward the midline of the body	Decreased
Abduction	Moving the extremity laterally and away from the midline of the body	Increased
Internal rotation	Rotating the extremity medially along its own axis	No change
External rotation	Rotating the extremity laterally along its own axis	No change
Circumduction	Moving the extremity in a conical fashion so that the distal aspect of the extremity moves in a circle	No change
Supination	Rotating the forearm laterally at the elbow so that the palm of the hand turns laterally to face upward	No change
Pronation	Rotating the forearm medially at the elbow so that the palm of the hand turns medially to face downward	No change
Opposition	Moving the thumb outward to touch the little finger of the same hand	No change
Inversion	Tilting the foot inward, with the medial side of the foot lowered	No change
Eversion	Tilting the foot outward, with the lateral side of the foot lowered	No change
Dorsiflexion	Flexing the foot at the ankle so that the toes move toward the chest	Decreased
Plantar flexion	Moving the foot at the ankle so that the toes move away from the chest	Increased
Elevation	Raising a body part in an upward direction	No change
Depression	Lowering a body part	No change
Protraction	Moving a body part anteriorly along its own axis (parallel to the ground)	No change
Retraction	Moving a body part posteriorly along its own axis (parallel to the ground)	No change
Gliding	One joint surface moves over another joint surface in a circular or angular nature	No change

lifestyle, and paralysis influence muscle tone. Identify muscle landmarks in arms and legs. Note any involuntary muscle movements, which may suggest adverse effects from medication (as in tardive dyskinesia) (see Chapter 13) or neurological system pathologies (see Chapter 12). Refer to Table 11-5 for types of involuntary movements.

Specific Musculoskeletal Assessment

Observe the contour of the joint and surrounding tissue. The joint should be rounded in flexion, and flat in extension. Tenderness, redness, swelling, or pain are abnormal findings. Swollen joints suggest arthritis or gout, whereas joint deformity may indicate joint displacement or **subluxation,** a dislodgment of bone from joint.

Palpation of muscle surrounding the joint gauges muscle tone. Start with the surrounding area and note any tenderness, pain, swelling, or nodules. Grating or popping are abnormal findings. Deformities may suggest gout, rheumatoid arthritis, or generalized inflammation.

Movement of the limbs in "north-south-east-west" motion assesses ROM. Note limitations and strengths in the older person's ability to span the directions. Pain and **crepitus** should be noted. Do not push the client beyond her or his ROM span. **Degenerative joint disease (DJD)** and rheumatoid arthritis may significantly limit ROM.

Muscle strength is assessed similarly. It should be equal on left and right sides. There should be no involuntary muscle movements. CVA, malnutrition, and neurological disorders alter muscle strength.

Palpating the joint while asking the client to open, close, and move the jaw side to side tests the temporomandibular joint. Clicking upon opening the mouth is normal. Smooth movement from side to side is also within normal limits. Pain and crepitus warrant further investigation, as they may be related to arthritis, dislocation, or poorly fitting dentures.

The cervical spine is assessed by first standing behind the client and palpating the neck and spinous processes. Next, stand in front of the client and ask her or him to:

• Touch chin to chest
• Touch ears to left and right shoulder
• Look up at the ceiling

Finally, apply resistance while performing the above tasks. Progressive DJD and arthritis will limit the client's ability to perform these tasks with or without resistance.

The shoulders are assessed by first standing in front of the client and observing for symmetry, shape, and size. Next palpate the scapula, shoulder, and surrounding muscles and sternoclavicular joint. Identify and palpate the acromion process, humerus, and biceps groove. No swelling, pain, or nodules should be found.

Testing the ROM of the shoulders is performed by moving the arms in the following directions:

• Forward arc **(forward flexion)**
• Backward arc **(hyperextension)**
• From sides to over the head **(abduction)**
• From sides to beyond the midline **(adduction)**
• Hands behind back and reach to scapulae **(internal rotation)**
• Shrug shoulders (tests CN XI)
• Place hands behind the head **(external rotation)**

No fluid or crepitus should be found. Repeat shoulder assessment while applying resistance.

It is not uncommon to find ROM limitations in older individuals resulting from DJD, arthritis, or disuse. With progressive stretching, ROM functions may be partially restored.

While standing at the side of the client, observe the elbows while the client flexes and extends them. Palpate the elbow and note the grooves at the **olecranon processes.** Ask the client to extend the arms with palms toward the ceiling and then toward the floor. Test strength by grasping the client's wrist and asking him

Table 11-4 Examples of Abnormal Gait Patterns

Type of Abnormal Gait	Etiology	Description
Antalgic	Degenerative joint disease of the hip or knee	Limited weight bearing is placed on an effected leg in an attempt to limit discomfort.
Short leg	Discrepancy in leg length, flexion contracture of the hip or knee, congenital hip dislocation	A limp is present during ambulation unless shoes have been adapted to compensate for length discrepancy.
Spastic hemiplegia	Cerebral palsy, unilateral upper motor neuron lesion (e.g., stroke)	Extension of one lower extremity with plantar flexion and foot inversion; arm is flexed at the elbow, wrist, and fingers. The patient walks by swinging the affected leg in a semicircle. The foot is not lifted off the floor. The affected arm does not swing with the gait.
Scissors	Multiple sclerosis, bilateral upper motor neuron disease	Adduction at the knee level produces short, slow steps. Gait is uncoordinated, stiff, and jerky. the foot is dragged across the floor in a semicircle.
Cerebellar ataxia	Cerebellar disease	Gait is broad based and uncoordinated, and the patient appears to stagger and sway during ambulation.
Sensory ataxia	Disorders of peripheral nerves, dorsal roots, and posterior column that watches the floor carefully interfere with proprioceptive input	Stance is broad based. Patient lifts feet up too high and abruptly slaps them on the floor, heel first. Help ensure correct foot placement because the patient is unaware of position in space.
Festinating	Parkinson's disease	Decreased step height and length, but increased step speed, resulting in "shuffling" (feet barely clearing the floor). Patient's posture is stooped and patient appears to hesitate both in initiation and in termination of ambulation. Rigid body position, with flexion of the knees during standing and ambulation.

Table 11-4 (continued)

Type of Abnormal Gait	Etiology	Description
Steppage or footdrop	Peroneal nerve injury, paralysis of the dorsiflexor muscles, damage to spinal nerve roots L5 and S1 from poliomyelitis	Hip and knee flexion are needed for step height in order to lift the foot off the floor. Instead of placing the heel of the foot on the floor first, the whole sole of the foot is slapped on the floor at once. May be unilateral or bilateral.
Apraxic	Alzheimer's disease, frontal lobe tumors	Patient has difficulty with walking despite intact motor and sensory systems. The patient is unable to initiate walking, as if stuck to the floor. After walking is initiated, the gait is slow and shuffling.
Trendelenburg	Developmental dysplasia of hip, muscular dystrophy	During ambulation, pelvis of the unaffected side drops when weight bearing is performed on the affected side. When both hips are affected, a "waddling" gait may be evident.

Table 11-5   Involuntary Muscle Movements

Type	Description
Fasciculation	Visible twitching of a group of muscle fibers that may be stimulated by the tapping of a muscle.
Fibrillation	Ineffective, uncoordinated muscle contraction that resembles quivering.
Spasm	Sudden muscle contraction. A cramp is a muscle spasm that is strong and painful. Clonic muscle spasms are contractions that alternate with a period of muscle relaxation. A tonic muscle spasm is a sustained contraction with a period of relaxation.
Tetany	Paroxysmal tonic muscle spasms, usually of the extremities. The face and jaw may also be affected by spasm. Tetany may be associated with discomfort.
Chorea	Rapid, irregular, and jerky muscle contractions of random muscle groups. It is unpredictable and without purpose. It can involve the face, upper trunk, and limbs. Sometimes, the patient tries to incorporate the movement into voluntary movement, which may appear grotesque and exaggerated. The patient may have difficulty with chewing, speaking, and swallowing.
Tremors	A period of continuous shaking due to muscle contractions. Although the quality of the tremors will be influenced by the cause, the amplitude and the frequency should remain the same. Tremors may be fine or coarse, rapid or slow, continuous or intermittent. They may be exacerbated during rest and attempts at purposeful movements, or by certain body positions.
Tic	Sudden, rapid muscle spasms of the upper trunk, face, or shoulders. The action is often repetitive and may decrease during purposeful movement. It can be persistent or limited in nature.
Ballism	Jerky, twisting movements due to strong muscle contraction.
Athetosis	Slow, writhing, twisting type of movement. The patient is unable to sustain any part of the body in one position. The movements are most often in the fingers, hands, face, throat, and tongue, although any part of the body can be affected. The movements are generally slower than in chorea.
Dystonia	Similar to athetosis but differing in the duration of the postural abnormality, and involving large muscles such as the trunk. The patient may present with an overflexed or overextended posture of the hand, pulling of the head to one side, torsion of the spine, inversion of the foot, or closure of the eyes and a fixed grimace.
Nyoclonus	A rapid, irregular contraction of a muscle or group of muscles, such as the type of jerking movement that occurs when drifting off to sleep.
Tremors at rest	Asymmetrical and coarse movements that disappear or diminish with action. They tend to diminish or cease with purposeful movement.

Table 11-5 (continued)	
Type	**Description**
Action tremors	Symmetrical or asymmetrical movements that increase in states of fatigue, weakness, drug withdrawal, hypocalcemia, uremia, or hepatic disease. This type of tremor may be induced in normal individuals when they are required to maintain a posture that demands extremes of power or precision. Action tremors are also called postural tremors.
Intention tremors	These tremors may appear only on voluntary movement of a limb and may intensify on termination of movement.
Asterixis	This is a variant of a tremor. The rate of limb flexion and extension is irregular, slow, and wide amplitude. The outstretched limb temporarily loses muscle tone.

or her to pull toward his or her chest while applying resistance. Red, warm, and swollen elbows may indicate gouty arthritis, bursitis, or rheumatoid arthritis.

Wrists and hands are assessed by inspecting for shape, position, and contour of fingers and wrist. Palpate each metacarpophalangeal joint, and each proximal and distal interphalangeal joint. Assess ROM of the wrists by asking the client to raise wrists to the ceiling (hyperextension) and lower them to the floor (flexion). Ask the client to touch each finger with the thumb of the same hand. With the wrist and forearm on a flat surface, secure the forearm and ask the client to "fight" against your resistance. The strength of the fingers is assessed by asking the client to push fingers together while you apply resistance. Ask the client to make a fist and release. If there are problems with strength and deformities, the client will have difficulty making a fist and fighting against resistance.

Test hand grasp by asking the client to squeeze your index and middle finger together as hard as possible. Grasps should be equal and strong.

Heberden's nodes, enlargement of the distal interphalangeal joints, are common findings in older people with osteoarthritis, caused by ankylosis and atrophy of the soft surrounding tissue. Pain may or may not be present.

NURSING TIP

Collaboration with the **occupational therapist** or **physical therapist** may be needed when deformities of the hand create inability to hold eating utensils, brush or comb, or a scissors. The occupational therapist's role is essential to gain depth in understanding and correcting deficits in activities of daily living. Physical therapists focus on mobility and risk of falls.

Assess the hips by inspecting and palpating landmarks. Identify the iliac crests for symmetry. While the client is aligned in a supine position, palpate the hip joints. Ask the client to perform the following tasks on each leg:

• Raise leg straight while the other leg remains on the exam table
• Raise leg to chest while leg is flexed at knee **(Thomas Test);** other leg is straight on exam table
• With leg flexed at the knee, move leg first medially, then laterally with foot outward/medially
• Swing straightened leg toward midline (adduction), then away from midline (abduction)
• While on abdomen (prone), lift leg

back with pelvis on the exam table (hyperextension)

Assess the strength of the hips by asking the client to do the following:

- Raise leg against the nurse's resistance on the anterior thigh above the knee
- Lower leg against the nurse's resistance behind and above the knee
- Move legs apart and together while the nurse applies resistance laterally and medially

If the client feels pain, a hip fracture may be present. Flexion contracture of the hip may surface when the client is unable to bring knee to chest while keeping the other leg on the exam table.

⚡ NURSING ALERT

Falls in older adults are known to increase nursing home admissions, deplete health care dollars, and, most important, increase mortality in older people. Prevention through assessment is critical.

Inspect the contour of the knees, which should appear smooth with some induration around the patella and should be aligned symmetrically. Palpate the surrounding muscles of the anterior thigh (quadriceps). Palpate the patella and suprapatellar pouch. Flex the client's knee 90 degrees to palpate the tibiofemoral joints; with thumbs on the anterior knee and fingers wrapped posteriorly, press in with the thumbs to palpate the tibial margins. Assess ROM by asking the client to perform the following:

- Bend and straighten knees
- Bend each knee while the nurse ap-

plies resistance under the knee and over the ankle

Inspecting for alignment and symmetry while walking and sitting assess the ankles, feet, and toes. Palpate the ankles and feet. Identify the Achilles tendon. Palpate each of the metatarsophalangeal joints. Ask the client to perform the following:

- Point toes toward chest, floor, outward and inward
- Curl toes, spread toes, move them together
- Point toes toward chest and spread toes while the nurse applies resistance

Note exaggerated arch, flat foot (pes planus), or bunion, all of which affect walking.

Assess the spine first by observing the individual posteriorly and laterally. Draw an imaginary line as indicated in Figures 11-3 (A and B).

Palpate the **spinal processes** with the thumb. Test ROM by asking the client to perform the following:

- Bend forward
- Bend side to side
- Bend backwards
- The nurse twists shoulders side to side

Abnormalities of the spine are depicted in Figure 11-4A, B, C, and D.

Functional Assessment

A reliable and accurate functional assessment is of prime importance in the older person. Functional status translates physiological, cognitive, and social findings into actual activities of daily living, which are essential to quality of life and well-being. Even though a person may have numerous medical diagnoses, she or he may still be able to carry out key functions as part of everyday living. Chronic illnesses tend to erode **ADLs (activities of daily living)** and **IADLs (instrumental activities of daily living)** and thus require special interdisciplinary problem-solving to pro-

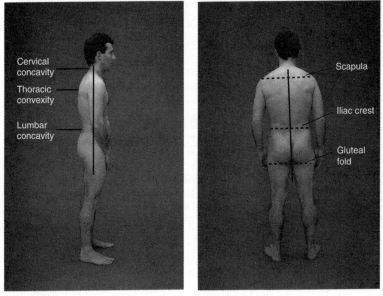

(A) Lateral view   (B) Posterior view

Figure 11-3   Alignment of Spinal Landmarks

mote optimal functioning and prevent functional decline. Although there are several functional assessment instruments, two have been selected for their usefulness and widespread use. In the Appendix are the Katz Index of Independence in Activities of Daily Living, as presented by The Hartford Institute for Geriatric Nursing, New York University; and the IADL assessment scale (Lawton & Brody, 1969). Although socioeconomic and environmental assessments are other dimensions contributing to functionality, they are incorporated in Chapter 3.

Table 11-6 shows characteristics of ADL and IADLs.

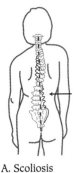
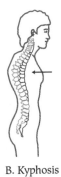
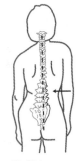

A. Scoliosis   B. Kyphosis   C. Lordosis   D. List

Figure 11-4   Abnormalities of the Spine

Table 11-6   ADLs and IADLs

ADLs skills	IADLs
Bathing	Telephone use
Dressing and grooming	Shopping
Toileting activities (use of toilet room, cleansing self after)	Ability to take medications
Transferring	Dishwashing, bed-making, house-cleaning, doing laundry
Feeding	Food preparation
Continence: bowel and bladder control	Managing transportation, whether walking, driving, or taking public transportation (subway, bus, cab)
Communication and cognition	Money management
Motivation to carry out ADLs	Motivation to carry out IADLs

*Note the difference between ADLs and IADLs: 'foundation' skills versus community-relatedness skills.

References

Cauthorne-Burnette, T., & Estes, M. E. Z., (1998). *Clinical companion for health assessment and physical examination.* Albany, NY: Delmar Publishers.

Shelkey, M., & Wallace, M. (1998). Katz Index of Independence in Activities of Daily Living (ADL). From *Best practices in nursing care to older adults, 1(2).* New York: The Hartford Institute for Geriatric Nursing, Division of Nursing.

Lawton, H. P., & Brody, E. M. (1969). Assessment of older people: Self-maintaining and instrumental activities of daily living. *Gerontologist, 9,* 179.

Matteson, M., McConnell, E. S., & Linton, A. D. (1997). *Gerontological nursing: Concepts and practice.* Philadelphia: W. B. Saunders.

12

Neurological Assessment

Key Terms

anesthesia
astereognosis
autonomic nervous system
central nervous system
cranial nerves
deep tendon reflexes (DTR)
dysesthesia
Glasgow Coma Scale
hyperesthesia
hypoesthesia
hypogeusia
hypothalamus
level of consciousness (LOC)
orientation
parasympathetic nervous system
paresthesia
pathological reflexes
peripheral nervous system
plantar reflex
pronator drift
stereoagnosis
superficial reflexes
sympathetic nervous system
thalamus
vertigo

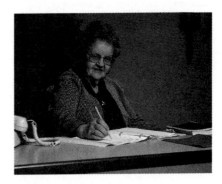

TIPS FROM THE EXPERTS

Individuals may feel like they have 'failed' when they are
unable to answer questions or perform certain skills. It is
paramount to reinforce that they are not competing with
anyone and that their inability is something they may be
able to improve on. The gerontological nurse and older
person work together to find the best ways to compensate
for neurological differences.

The neurological assessment is complex, especially in older adults. The nervous system is an intricate network comprised of computer "hard drive" (the brain), the "electrical cables" (spinal cord), and localized sets of "software" (neuronal networks). All are interrelated and coordinated to carry out basic life functions such as heartbeat and respiration, voluntary movement, and thought processes. Figures 12-1 and 12-2 and Table 12-1 depict brain anatomy, spinal cord, and cranial nerves.

Central and Peripheral Nervous Systems

Characteristics of both the central and peripheral nervous systems are outlined in Tables 12-2 and 12-3.

Age-Related Neurological Changes

Table 12-4 summarizes age-related changes in the neurological functioning in older people. As part of the health history, note medical diagnoses such as cerebral aneurysm, stroke, migraines, Alzheimer's disease, or seizures. Medications such as psychotropics and antidepressessants also affect individuals neurologically.

Neurological Assessment Techniques

There are six dimensions to the neurological assessment:

- Assessment of mental status (see Chapter 13)

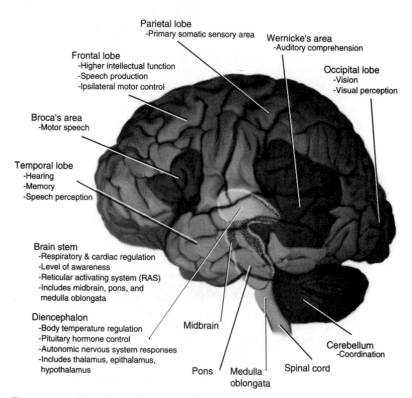

Figure 12-1 Locations and functions of the cerebral lobes, brain stem, and cerebellum

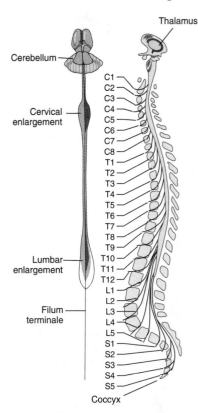

Thalamus

Cerebellum

Cervical enlargement

Lumbar enlargement

Filum terminale

C1
C2
C3
C4
C5
C6
C7
C8
T1
T2
T3
T4
T5
T6
T7
T8
T9
T10
T11
T12
L1
L2
L3
L4
L5
S1
S2
S3
S4
S5
Coccyx

Figure 12-2 Spinal cord and spinal nerves

- Sensation (see Chapter 7)
- Cranial nerves (CN)
- Motor function
- Cerebellar function
- Reflexes

Table 12-5 offers a quick neurological reference useful for screening areas in need of greater assessment depth.

Types of aphasia are described in Table 12-6.

Level of Consciousness

Level of consciousness (LOC) is the term used to describe the degree of wakefulness and alertness of a person. LOC is determined through observation, assessment of verbal response, and assessment of motor responses.

Table 12-1   Functions of the Cranial Nerves

Name and Number	Function
Olfactory (I)	Smell
Optic (II)	Visual acuity, visual fields, funduscopic examination
Oculomotor (III)	Cardinal fields of gaze (EOM movement), eyelid elevation, pupil reaction, doll's eyes phenomenon
Trochlear (IV)	EOM movement
Trigeminal (V)	Motor: strength of temporalis and masseter muscles Sensory: light touch, superficial pain, temperature to face, corneal reflex
Abducens (VI)	EOM movement
Facial (VII)	Motor: facial movements Sensory: taste anterior two-thirds of tongue *Parasympathetic: tears and saliva secretion
Acoustic (VIII)	Cochlear: gross hearing, Weber and Rinne tests Vestibular: vertigo, equilibrium, nystagmus
Glossopharyngeal (IX)	Motor: soft palate and uvula movement, gag reflex, swallowing, guttural and palatal sounds Sensory: taste posterior one-third of tongue *Parasympathetic: carotid reflex, chemoreceptors
Vagus (X)	Motor and Sensory: same as CN IX *Parasympathetic: carotid reflex, stomach and intestinal secretions, peristalsis, involuntary control of bronchi, heart innervation
Spinal Accesory (XI)	Sternocleidomastoid and trapezius muscle movements
Hyposglossal (XII)	Tongue movement, lingual sounds

Cannot be directly assessed.
EOM = extraocular muscle; CN = cranial nerve.

Notice how the client reacts to the environment. Is the client comfortable in the environment? Anxious? Hostile? Distracted? Any unusual responses may indicate neurological and/or other problems. Difficulty following verbal requests may be due to pathology.

If the client is not alert and responsive, it may be necessary to test for response to painful stimuli. This is done by pressing down on the fingernail bed or pinching the trapezius muscle. The **Glasgow Coma Scale** is a well known scale used to determine LOC. A score of 15 indicates full alertness based on totals of the three categories. See Figure 12-3.

Orientation to person, place, and time traditionally has been used to assess orientation to reality. A client who is oriented should be able to verbalize her name, name of a significant other, where she is and where she lives, date, and time. Date

Table 12-2 The Central Nervous System

Central Nervous System (brain and spinal cord)
- Cerebrum (right and left)
  - Cerebral cortex (outer layer): memory storage and recall; sensation
- Diencephalon
  - Thalamus: controls sensory stimuli except olfactory; pain, touch, temperature sensation
  - Epithalamus: includes pineal body (melatonin synthesis)
  - Hypothalamus: controls metabolism, water balance, body temperature
- Cerebellum
  - Two lobes: control movement
  - Vermis: midportion; controls equilibrium
- Brain stem
  - Midbrain
    - CN III (oculomotor) [see section on cranial nerves]
    - CN IV (trochlear)
  - Pons
    - CN V (trigeminal)
    - CN VI (abducens)
    - CN VII (facial)
    - CN VIII (acoustic)
  - Medulla oblongata (extends into the spinal cord)
    - CN IX (glossopharyngeal)
    - CN X (vagus)
    - CN XI (spinal accessory)
    - CN XII (hypoglossal)

Adapted from Guyton, A. C., & Hall, J. E. (1996). *Textbook of medical physiology* (9th ed.). Philadelphia: W. B. Saunders Company.

and time may become less significant to older people who lack routine, structure in their lives, and purpose. As one older woman stated, "I don't have children to get on a school bus or a job to go to. So why do I have to know the day or time?" This older person poses an interesting challenge to nurses: What is the meaning

Table 12-3 The Peripheral Nervous System

Peripheral Nervous System (nerves peripheral to central nervous system):
- Spinal nerves (thirty-one pairs)
  - Eight cervical
  - Twelve thoracic
  - Five lumbar
  - One coccygeal
- Cranial nerves (twelve pairs)
- **Autonomic nervous system** (maintains vital functions "automatically" or involuntarily)
- **Sympathetic**
  - "fight or flight" survival mechanism to danger (i.e., increased heart rate, pupillary dilation, vasoconstriction)
- **Parasympathetic**
  - Stimulation includes slowed heart rate, smooth muscle contraction, bronchiole constriction, pupillary constriction

and value of reality orientation in some groups of older individuals?

Judgment and Insight

Judgment is tested by asking questions about situations requiring decision-making and problem-solving. Impaired judgment insinuates potential safety problems. Use questions such as:

- What would you do if your toaster caught on fire?
- What would you do if you had a flat tire? Power outage? Telephone failure?
- If you saw that another resident, neighbor, or visitor had fainted, what would you do?

Assess for logical problem-solving and reasoning. Does the answer the client offers make sense? Forms of dementia, depression, cognitive impairment, and psychological disorders tend to cloud judgment. Cognitive status and differences

Table 12-4   Summary of Age-Related Neurological Changes

- Brain decreases in size (by approximately 7 percent)
- Loss of neurons in the brain (up to 20 percent)
- Possible decrease in cerebral blood flow
- Little decline in intellect
- Increase in serotonin, decrease in norepinephrine (possibly contributes to depression)
- Slowing in deep tendon reflexes
- Slowing in peripheral nerve conduction
- Decreased speed of motor coordination
- Overall decrease in autonomic and sympathetic nervous system functions
- **Hypothalamus** function: decreased control of thermoregulation
- Some memory changes:
- Losses in short-term memory
- Clarity of long-term memory
- Some difficulty learning new information and retaining it; holds implications for client teaching about medications, procedures, prevention, etc.

Summarized from Matteson, M., McConnell, E. S., & Linton, A. D. (1997). *Gerontological nursing: Concepts and practice*. Philadelphia: W. B. Saunders Company.

among dementia, depression, and delirium are covered in Chapter 13.

Sensation and Sensory Assessment

Examine Chapter 7. In addition, the procedures and findings for sensory assessment are illustrated in Table 12-7.

Cranial Nerves

How each cranial nerve is tested is listed in Table 12-8.

Motor System

See Chapter 11 for musculoskeletal assessment. Rigidity in muscle movement may indicate extrapyramidal agitation, Parkinson's disease, or basal ganglia lesions. Test for **pronator drift.** Have the client close eyes, extend arms with palms up for 30 seconds. If one arm tends to drift downward, a stroke is suggested.

🖋 NURSING ALERT

Risk Factors for Stroke

Significant risk factors for stroke include:

- Hypertension
- Diabetes mellitus
- Cocaine use
- Cigarette smoking
- Hyperlipidemia
- Chronic atrial fibrillation and flutter
- Sickle cell disease
- IV drug abuse
- Alcohol abuse
- Obesity
- Oral contraceptive use, especially in women who are over age 35 and who smoke and have hypertension

---

Cerebellar Function

Ask the client to:

- touch nose with index finger and then touch the opposite index finger, repeating this motion several times. Ask the client to repeat this with eyes closed.
- (eyes opened) to touch nose with index finger, then to touch your index finger while you change the position of your index finger. Repeat this procedure on the opposite side of the client.
- pat knees and rapidly change from palms up to palms down.
- touch thumb to each finger (of the same hand) rapidly. Repeat with both hands.
- slide heel up and down side of the opposite leg. Repeat on opposite side
- draw a figure 8 with one foot in the air. Repeat with opposite foot.

Table 12-5 Neurological Screening Assessment

Assessment Parameter	Assessment Skill	Comments
Mental status/ and sensory assessment.	Note general appearance, affect, speech content, memory, logic, judgment, and speech patterns during the history.	If any abnormalities or inconsistencies are evident, perform full mental status assessment.
	Perform Glasgow Coma Scale (GCS) with motor assessment component and pupil assessment.	IF GCS < 15, perform full assessment of mental status and consciousness. If motor assessment is abnormal or asymmetrical, perform complete motor and sensory assessment
Sensation	Assess pain and vibration in the hands and feet, light touch on the limbs.	If deficits are identified, perform a complete sensory assessment.
Cranial nerves	Assess CN II, III< IV, VI: visual acuity gross visual fields, funduscopic examination, pupillary reactions, and extraocular movements. Assess CN VII, VII, IX, X, XII: facial expression, gross hearing, voice and tongue.	If any abnormalities exist, perform complete assessment of all twelve cranial nerves.
Motor system	• Muscle tone and strength • Abnormal movements • Grasps	If deficits are noted, perform a complete motor system assessment.

Cerebellar function	Observe the client's:
	1. Gait on arrival
	2. Ability to:
	  • Walk heel-to-toe • Hop in place
	  • Walk on toes • Perform shallow knee
	  • Walk on heels bends
	3. Check Romberg's sign.
		If any abnormalities exist, perform complete cerebellar assessment.

Reflexes	Assess the muscle stretch reflexes and the plantar response.	If an abnormal response is elicited, perform a complete reflex assessment.

Table 12-6 Classification of Aphasias

Aphasia	Pathophysiology	Expression	Characteristics
Broca's aphasia	Motor cortex lesion, Broca's area	Expressive Nonfluent	Speech slow and hesitant, the client has difficulty in selecting and organizing words. Naming, word and phrase repetition, and writing impaired. Subtle defects in comprehension.
Wernicke's aphasia	Left hemisphere lesion in Wernicke's area	Receptive Fluent	Auditory comprehension impaired, as is content of speech. Client unaware of deficits. Naming severely impaired.
Anomic aphasia	Left hemisphere lesion in Wernicke's area	Amnesic Fluent	Client unable to name objects or places. Comprehension and repetition of words and phrases intact.
Conduction aphasia	Lesion in the arcuate fasciculus, which connects and transports messages between Broca's and Wernicke's areas	Central Fluent	Client has difficulty repeating words, substitutes incorrect sounds for another (e.g., *dork* for *fork*).
Global aphasia	Lesions in the frontal-temporal area	Mixed Fluent	Both oral and written comprehension severely impaired, naming, repetition of words and phrases, ability to write impaired.
Transcortical sensory aphasia	Lesion in the periphery of Broca's and Wernicke's areas (watershed zone)	Fluent	Impairment in comprehension, naming, and writing. Word and phrase repetition intact.
Transcortical motor aphasia	Lesion anterior, superior, or lateral to Broca's area	Nonfluent	Comprehension intact. Naming and ability to write impaired. Word and phrase repetition intact.

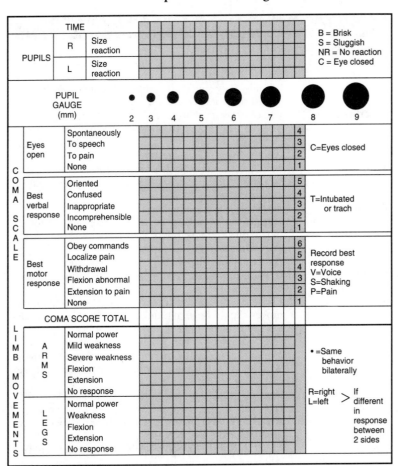

Figure 12-3 Neurological flow sheet, including Glasgow Coma Scale

- Flex and extend each foot separately and rapidly.

In all instances, smooth and coordinated motions should be noted; speed will vary with age.

Reflexes

Testing reflexes, right and left sides, assesses the speed and degree of response. A 0 to 4+ is the scale used to identify grading of reflexes. With the reflex hammer held loosely and with a quick strike to the tendon, response is assessed:

NURSING TIP

The neurologist specializes in knowledge and treatment of neurological system disorders. The focus is usually on nonsurgical, pharmacological interventions.

- 0 = absent
- 1+ = diminished response
- 2+ = normal
- 3+ = somewhat increased (not pathological)

Table 12-7   Exteroceptive, Proprioceptive, and Cortical Sensation

*conducted with client's eyes closed

Light touch	Client says 'yes' when sensation is felt; wisp of cotton ball brushed over hands, arms, abdomen, leg, foot, bilaterally. Vary speed and pattern. Identify areas of impaired sensation.
Superficial pain	Use object with sharp and dull side. Client says "dull" or "sharp" when sensation is felt. Sites are same as above. *Do not* press sharp object deeply into the skin! Identify areas of impaired sensation.
Temperature	Tested for if above findings are abnormal. Client says "warm" or "cold" as test tubes of each liquid is placed at above sites.
Responses to light touch, pain, temperature	**Anesthesia** (cannot feel touch) **Hypoesthesia** or **hyperesthesia** (feels little or too much touch/pain sensation) **Paresthesia** (numbness, tingling) **Dyesthesia** (inability to distinguish sensations)
Possible problems	Lesions or breakdown of nerves, **thalamus,** upper brainstem
Motion	Client says "up," "down" or "can't tell" when the nurse moves client's fingers in those directions. Inability suggests thalamus or peripheral neuropathies.
Vibration	Client says "yes" when vibration is felt. Place vibrating tuning fork on boney prominences (ankle, toe, finger, wrist, elbow). Polyneuropathies are common in those over 65 years old.
Cortical sensation	**Stereoagnosis** (knowing objects by touch) Hand client a pen or watch. Ask client to identify it. **Astereognosis** (unable to name object by touch) suggests parietal lobe problems.
Two-point discrimination	Client says "two" or "one" as two sharp points are felt when touched simultaneously at the fingertips, feet, truck, 0.5 centimeters apart. Inability suggests parietal lobe problems.
Extinction	Client says "one" or "two" when cotton-tipped applicators are placed at same sites on the body, then one is removed. Inability suggests parietal lobe problems.

NURSING TIP

There are three categories of reflexes: **deep tendon reflexes (DTR), superficial reflexes,** and **pathological reflexes.** Testing the reflexes tests the speed and appropriate response of nerve conduction based on stimulation. The responses are documented based on the three categories.

Table 12-8 Testing Each Cranial Nerve

Cranial nerve	How each is tested
CN I (olfactory nerve)	Client (eyes closed) smells different odors, each nostril separately. Two quick, deep breaths are taken. Garlic, cinnamon, and coffee may be used. Compare differences between nostrils.
CN II (optic nerve)	See Chapter 7 on visual acuity and visual fields.
CN III (oculomotor nerve)	See Chapter 7 on cardinal fields of gaze and eyelid elevation. Test pupillary reaction.
CN IV (trochlear nerve)	See Chapter 7 on cardinal fields of gaze.
CN V (trigeminal nerve)	Client clenches jaw and moves jaw from side to side while nurse palpates contraction of temporalis and masseter muscles. Symmetry and moderate strength are normal findings. (See Figures 12-4A and B.)
CN VI (abducens nerve)	Cardinal fields of gaze (see Chapter 7).
CN VII (facial nerve)	A. Client frowns, raises eyebrows, smiles, shows teeth, purses lips, puffs out cheeks while nurse applies resistance. Examine symmetry and strength. B. Test taste. Nurse places sweet and salty substance at tip of tongue with cotton-tipped applicator; sour substance at tip and borders; back of tongue and soft palate for bitter. Client rinses mouth between applications. **Hypogeusia** (reduced taste sensation) is common with aging.
CN VIII (acoustic nerve)	Hearing and Weber & Rinne tests (Chapter 7). Ask about presence of **vertigo** (sense of movement in the environment).
CN IX and CN X (glossopharyngeal and vagus nerves)	Test gag reflex (Chapter 7). Test swallow reflex (swallowing a small amount of water). Test sounds: *k, q, ch, b, d*. Test CN VII (posterior one-third of tongue) as indicated. Abnormalities comprise: nasal vocal qualities, inability to taste, and dysphagia.
CN XI (spinal accessory nerve)	Test bilateral facial muscles. Place resistance with hand on left and right sides of face, asking client to resist and turn face in opposite direction. Inspect and palpate sternocleidomastoid muscle. Next ask client to raise shoulders while applying resistance. Compare strength.
CN XII (hypoglossal nerve)	See Chapter 7. Tongue movement. Lingual speech is noted as clear.

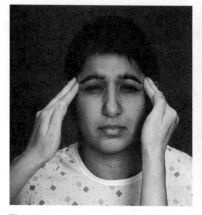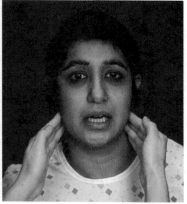

Figure 12-4   Motor component of CN V

- 4+ = very increased, clonus may be present

Points of stimulation/tapping are shown in Figures 12-5A through E. These include biceps, brachioradialis, triceps, patella, and achilles.

Losses in reflexes suggest coma, drug sedation, intracranial pressure, impaired cortex function, pyramidal dysfunction, tetany, or tetanus.

Testing superficial reflexes requires three procedures. First, with the client lying down, abdomen exposed, elicit the abdominal reflex by 'criss-crossing' the abdomen above the umbilicus with the opposite end of a cotton-tipped applicator. Observe for abdominal contraction during

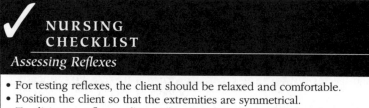

✓ **NURSING CHECKLIST**

Assessing Reflexes

- For testing reflexes, the client should be relaxed and comfortable.
- Position the client so that the extremities are symmetrical.
- To elicit true reflexes, distract the client by talking about another topic.
- Loosely hold the reflex hammer between the thumb and index finger and use a brisk motion from the wrist to strike the tendon. The reflex hammer should make contact with the correct point on the tendon in a quick, direct manner.
- Observe the degree and speed of response of the muscles after the reflex hammer makes contact. Grading of reflexes is as follows:
    - 0: absent
    - + (1+): present but diminished
    - ++ (2+): normal
    - +++ (3+): mildly increased but not pathological
    - ++++ (4+): markedly hyperactive, clonus may be present
- Compare reflex responses of the right and left sides. Taps in the correct area should elicit a brisk (i.e., 2+ or 3+) contraction of the muscles involved.

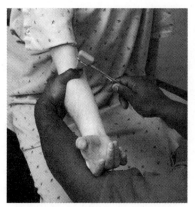

A. Biceps

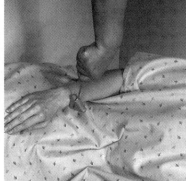

B. Brachioradialis

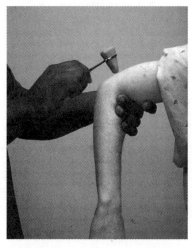

C. Triceps

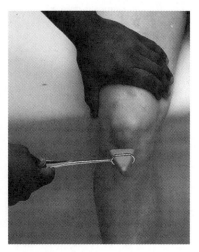

D. Patellar

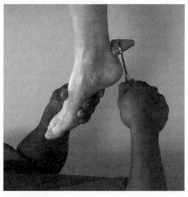

E. Achilles

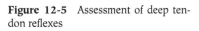

Figure 12-5   Assessment of deep tendon reflexes

each motion. Then repeat this procedure below the umbilicus in the lower abdominal quadrants. Contraction should be noted in response to the stimulus.

To test for the **plantar reflex,** stroke the outer and underside of the foot with the handle of the reflex hammer. Some degree of flexion is normal.

Responses of the cremasteric and bulbocavernosus muscles are tested for in men. While the male client is lying down, stroke the inner thigh (one side at a time), above and downward at the level of the groin. Contraction of the cremasteric muscle should be noted. When the skin of the foreskin or glans penis is pinched, the perineum at the base of the penis should contract (bulbocavernosus muscle).

Be mindful that many of these procedures are quite intrusive and must be preceded by clear explanation.

References

Cathorne-Burnette, T., & Zator Estes, M. (1998). *Clinical companion for health assessment and physical examination.* Albany: Delmar Publishers.

Guyton, A. C., & Hall, J. E. (1996). *Textbook of medical physiology* (9th ed.). Philadelphia: W. B. Saunders Company.

Matteson, M., McConnell, E. S., & Linton, A. D. (1997). *Gerontological nursing: Concepts and practice.* Philadelphia: W. B. Saunders Company.

13

Mental Health Assessment

Key Terms

affective
cognition
delirium
dementia
depression
psychotropics
polypharmacy
self-esteem
self-neglect
sleep apnea
social skills
tardive dyskinesia

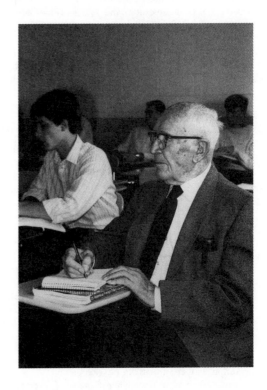

TIPS FROM THE EXPERTS

Suicide can be overlooked in older people. The presence of any of the following factors should alert the nurse: living alone, male, Caucasian, sense of hopelessness, advanced age (over 85). In addition, history of prior suicide attempts, family history of suicide, and substance abuse are "red flags" for predicting suicide attempts.

Assessment of an individual's level of mental health requires a holistic approach. It is somewhat different than conducting a cardiovascular assessment, for example. Unlike auscultating heart sounds, mental health assessment calls forth a different set of nursing skills. The stethoscope is a vital instrument in the cardiovascular assessment. Likewise, the nurse's skillfulness in observation, communication, and understanding of human behavior with strong psychological and sociological underpinnings become the tools used in the mental status assessment of an older adult.

One potential pitfall in mental status assessment is arriving at premature and often erroneous clinical conclusions. Scheduling several sessions with the older adult may prevent this from happening. Upon the initial meeting with the older adult, it is not uncommon to observe behaviors reflecting anxiety. Because of fear, insecurity, lack of confidence, suspiciousness of health care personnel, or previously negative experiences with nurses, an older adult may initially be anxious. It is the nurse's responsibility to create a comfort level through establishing rapport. Appropriate use of touch, some "small talk," plus perhaps having a family member present (if the older adult is agreeable) tend to reduce tension and dispel fear.

If after several sessions with the older adult the anxiety persists, then a *pattern of behavior* is present. When patterns are identified, the nurse asks why these are occurring. Is there a possible physiological cause, such as an underlying disease? Is the behavior consistent with a medication reaction? Has the older adult experienced a crisis event recently that may have precipitated the behavior? After possible physiological roots or causes are explored, then and *only then* are psychological causes pursued and nursing diagnoses established.

A wide variety of psychological testing instruments screen for **affective** (mood) and **cognitive** (thought) problems. Regardless of the tests used, the basics include the keen observations of physical appearance, movements and body language, affect, clarity of thought processes, and orientation to surroundings and reality/time, all within the cultural context of the individual and within the existing environment. In addition, eating and sleeping patterns are explored because changes may reflect symptoms of changes in mental health. During the initial comprehensive or episodic health history with the older adult, the nurse formulates impressions of behavior. An awareness of some of the influences on the mental health of older adults provides the knowledge necessary to help understand some of the observed behaviors.

Age-Related Changes and Mental Health

It is difficult to directly connect physiological changes with changes in mental functioning. There is not a clear cause-effect relationship. In other words, we are unable to say that a loss of one hundred neurons will cause mild memory loss. Likewise, a two hundred neuron loss cannot necessarily be equated with moderate memory loss. Neurologically, the body manages to *adapt* and *compensate* for cellular changes and deterioration. Table 13-1 lists physiological age-related changes associated with thought processes and memory. Table 13-2 shows psychosocial and spiritual influences that are often associated with the aging population.

Components of Mental Assessment

Mental assessment underlies the complete or episodic health history, or for that matter, any nursing interaction with an older adult. First impressions are recorded, and include an objective description of the initial greeting, handshake, use of language, appropriateness of clothing, and ability to socialize **(social skills)**. Often but not always when personal care is lacking, **self-esteem** or **self-neglect** is in question. If someone else such as a family member, nursing assistant, or home health aide

Table 13-1 Suspected Physiological Factors Related to Mental Health Changes in the Older Adult

- Decrease in large neurons
- Decrease in brain volume and brain weight
- Some decrease in short-term memory; long-term memory stays about the same
- Increase in reaction time to external stimuli
- Mild changes in sense of spatial accuracy and spatial relationships

Summarized from Burke, M., & Walsh, M. (1997). *Gerontologic nursing: Wholistic care of the older adult.* St Louis: Mosby-Year Book, Inc.

meets the older adult's personal needs, other deductions are made about mental health.

In the nursing home setting, where a resident may be bathed, dressed, and groomed by the certified nursing assistant (CNA), it is expected that the resident will appear clean, neat, and appropriate in ap-

Table 13-2 Suspected Psychosocial and Spiritual Factors Associated with Mental Health in the Older Adult

- Multiple losses (loss of youth, loss of spouse, home, family, job, income)
- Loneliness versus sense of connection to others
- Hopelessness versus hopefulness
- Fear of death versus sense of peace
- Low self-worth versus positive self-esteem
- Negative coping mechanisms; i.e., substance abuse
- Meaninglessness in life versus sense of purposefulness

pearance on a consistent basis. However, imagine a charge nurse on a nursing home unit. Upon examining the facial expression and posture of a nursing home resident, the nurse notices that the resident has a slumped posture, eyes are downcast, and the brow is furrowed with lack of attentiveness. In addition, the resident's arms are folded across her chest and her gait is sluggish. Several alternative explanations should be investigated: depression of the resident, abuse from the CNA, exacerbation of an existing illness, onset of a new illness, or medication dosage issues. This line of questioning and investigating is paramount not only to the assessment of mental health of an older adult, but also to the assessment of overall health. The behaviors listed in the example above are *not* considered within normal parameters and warrant further nursing intervention.

Movement and motor coordination in an older adult may appear stiff and slower than that of a younger adult. The walking stride in an older person is generally shorter and the stance is usually wider. Dexterity in skills such as tying shoes and writing may be diminished. In examining the older client, cautiousness in walking and in balance may be noted because of heightened consciousness in movement due to osteoarthritis, osteoporosis, or fear of falling. Some cautiousness is expected, yet if cautiousness becomes extreme and obsessive, an older adult may refuse to leave his or her home, leading to potential social isolation, loneliness, and even depression.

Odors emanating from the older adult's body and mouth should be noted. Physical illness, self-neglect resulting from some form of mental illness, or socioeconomic factors such as homelessness, poverty, and lack of access to health care should be investigated thoroughly.

Listen closely to the older adult's quality and quantity of speech and language. Are sentences complete? What is the amplitude of the speech? Is speech too loud? Too soft? Too rapid or slow? Does the person use slang? Does the person circumvent answering questions? Does the person perseverate (stay on the same topic and continue to return to it)? Is aphasia (speech impairment) present? Strokes, cranial nerve deficits, hearing problems, thyroid function abnormalities, substance abuse, and educational impairments are possible explanations for speech abnormalities. Table 13-3 reviews terms used in describing speech and language findings. Consult with a speech therapist for further explanation.

Body language and facial expression are other indicators of mental health or illness. Numerous books on body language have been written. Some principles may apply to older adults. For example, excessive "fidgeting" movements may be indicative of anxiety. On the other hand, they may indicate pain or a neurological disorder. A second example is degree of eye contact. When eye contact with the nurse is avoided, the nurse may hypothesize that the older adult is experiencing low self-esteem. Further interactions are necessary to support this by posing questions such as, "Describe yourself" or "Describe how you feel most of the time." It is important that the nurse consider cultural influences when examining degree of eye contact. Some cultures are not comfortable with making or maintaining eye contact.

Holding or folding arms across the chest usually sends the message that someone does not want to communicate or interact.

Similarly, the message of not wanting to receive the communication is also being displayed. Smiling, grimacing, frowning, unusual crying, giddiness, laughter, lip-biting, lip-smacking, or excessive facial movements all may indicate various problems such as mood swings, anxiety, depression, medication reaction, hyperthyroidism, stroke, or Parkinsonism, to name a few.

Never presume that mental illness is present based on physical appearance and first impressions of an older adult. As a more comprehensive physical and psychosocial examination unfolds so, too, will the data to support or refute presence of mental illness. Table 13-4 summarizes the components of the mental health assessment, highlighting keen observation and analytical skills of the nurse. Neurological assessment is covered in Chapter 12.

When lack of attention occurs, the nurse needs to ask what may be occurring. An older adult's inability to concentrate on tasks or interview questions may reflect a neurological deficit. In addition, observe and note aggressive or wandering behavior, often seen in dementia.

Sleeping patterns change as persons age. The major change is an increase in light sleep and a decrease in deep sleep, resulting in subjective perception of a less than restful sleep. Quality and quantity of

---

Table 13-3   Terminology Associated with Speech/Language Findings in Older Adults

- **Aphasia:** impairment of language
- **Apraxia:** inability to actually verbalize a word that is thought of in the mind
- **Alexia:** inability to understand the meaning of a word/sentences
- **Agraphia:** inability to write
- **Dysphonia:** a disorder of the larynx whereby a person in unable to make the sounds of a word(s)
- **Dysarthria:** lack of muscular control in mouth, face, neck, throat, or brain needed to speak
- **Circumlocution:** unable to answer a question: "circles around" the topic, but is unable to answer the question/topic
- **Confabulation:** when memory fails, a "making up " of answers

---

From Estes, M. E. Z. (1998). *Health assessment and physical examination* (Chapter 18). Albany, NY: Delmar Publishers.

Table 13-4 Components of Mental Assessment in the Older Adult

*Inspection and analysis are the two major skills used.

Observe for:

- Physical appearance, grooming, and dressing (*not* a parameter when personal needs are provided by others; i.e. in a nursing home setting)
- Cultural and educational background
- Posture
- Movement
- Body language
- Facial expression
- Level of alertness and attentiveness

Analyze:

- Sleeping and eating patterns
- Medication usage
- Psychiatric history
- Laboratory test results
- Results of standardized cognition, orientation, judgment, and reasoning and depression scales (*interpret cautiously; many of these screening tests have minimal clinical value for older adult populations)

---

sleep are assessed by asking the older adult if there has been a recent change in sleeping patterns:

- numbers of hours slept per night
- naps
- restfulness
- interruptions in sleep
- sleeping aids used

Exhaustion during the day may indicate **sleep apnea.** In fact, sleep deprivation mimics signs and symptoms of psychosis and mental illness, illustrating the importance of examining sleeping patterns.

A similar analysis of eating patterns is conducted. Besides reflecting nutritional status, changes in eating patterns and in appetite may indicate stress and mental problems. Overeating or undereating as a change in eating pattern associated with a life event or crisis strongly correlates with ineffective coping. Look for weight loss or gain as objective evidence, using the data to prompt further discussion with the older adult.

Examine connections among medications, laboratory test results, and medical diagnoses that may hold behavioral implications changes (i.e., hypothyroidism, COPD) and psychiatric diagnoses (i.e., depression, schizophrenia). The model from Chapter 3 (the triad of inquiry) will facilitate the thought process of analyzing data. The model as applied to assessing mental status might look like Figure 13-1. Areas in bold indicate clinical connections.

Medication use or misuse, multiple prescribing practitioners, **polypharmacy** (too many medications other than that which is needed), and cost of medications are examined relative to behavioral symptoms in the older adult. There are numerous medications, that may potentially alter the older adult's behavior and personality. Table 13-5 lists several medication categories and circumstances precipitating behavioral changes.

Cognition is part of the mental status assessment. Although standardized cognitive assessment tools may have limited value in testing older adults, especially those with moderate to severe cognitive impairment, formal testing is done to establish baseline data from which changes are measured. Formal testing is done:

- upon admission to the nursing home and periodically, usually every six months
- sometimes upon admission to a home care agency
- as clinically warranted when behavioral and personality changes are noted

The following section defines cognition and offers two cognitive scales and two depression scales.

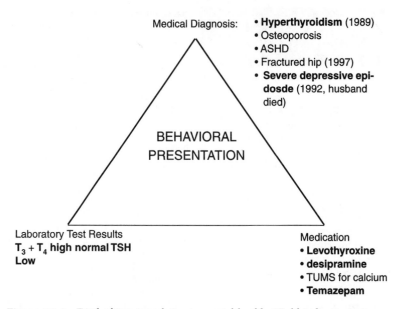

Medical Diagnosis: • **Hyperthyroidism** (1989)
• Osteoporosis
• ASHD
• Fractured hip (1997)
• **Severe depressive epidosde** (1992, husband died)

BEHAVIORAL
PRESENTATION

Laboratory Test Results
T_3 + T_4 high normal TSH Low

Medication
• **Levothyroxine**
• **desipramine**
• TUMS for calcium
• **Temazepam**

Figure 13-1   Triad of inquiry relative to mental health. *Bold indicates a strong connection.

Cognition

Cognition is a term used to describe the process by which people experience their world. It is the wholistic blend of perceiving the environment, interpreting it, and using logic and reasoning to maneuver through the world paired with utilizing judgment and memory to make everyday decisions. Clearly, cognition is a complex function integrating language and calculation skills, short- and long-term memory capacity skills, and spatial relationships.

In a healthy older adult, little cognitive changes occur. However, as pathological conditions surface, any or all of the aspects of cognition are altered. For example, the disease process of cerebrovascular accident (CVA, or stroke) from uncontrolled hypertension can result in poor safety judgment, memory and spatial difficulties, and speech impairments. Translated into everyday activities, activities of daily living (ADLS) or instrumental activities of daily living (IADLS) are likely to be affected:

• inability to select proper clothing
• difficulty using and remembering to turn the stove off
• forgetting to take medications
• inability to decide what to do if a fire occurred
• not knowing how to dial the telephone
• inability to know how to bathe, dress, or feed self

It is important to measure the degree to which cognition is impaired; guessing is dangerous. Individuals who have excellent social skills are adept at covering for cognitive losses. On the other hand, those who may be exceptionally quiet or timid do not readily demonstrate their cognitive abilities. Make no assumptions. If one of the standardized tools is not used, some rudimentary questions such as the ones below can help ascertain a problem with thought processes. If the person is unable to answer the questions below, cognition and memory may be impaired:

Table 13-5   Medication Categories and Side Effects That May Alter Behaviors in Older Adults

*Note that if a *nonpharmacological* intervention can be used to treat the problem, use as a first choice in lieu of medicating the older adult.

1. Anticholinergics:
   - General side effects: dry mouth, urinary retention, constipation, blurred vision, tachycardia, palpitations, aggravation of glaucoma, confusion
   - Diphenhydramine, atropine or derivative, some over-the-counter cold medications
2. Antianxiety agents (anxiolytics):
   - Anticholinergic effects: oversedation, lethargy, muscle relaxation, ataxia, paradoxical hyperactivity, restlessness, emotional outbursts, rage
   - Benzodiazepines: alprazolam, diazepam, lorazepam
3. Psychotropics, antidepressants (tricyclics):
   - Anticholinergic effects: orthostatic hypotension, oversedation, extrapyramidal symptoms, tremors, agitation, cardiotoxicity
   - Amantadine, carbamezepine, doxepin, desipramine, sertraline, flurazepam, lithium, and more
4. Sedative and hypnotics:
   - Hypotension, oversedation, lethargy, drowsiness, paradoxical effect of hyperactivity, increased fall risk, confusion, and disorientation
   - Benzodiazepines: temazepam, zolpidem
5. Anti-Parkinson's agents:
   - Extrapyramidal symptoms: tremors, abnormal muscle movements, akinesia
   - Anticholinergic effects: as above
   - Levodopa with carbidopa, diphenhydramine
6. Alcohol usage with the above drug categories enhances central nervous system (CNS) depression: sedation, lethargy, drowsiness
7. Any drug in too large a dose: overdose, toxicity symptoms, and delirium
8. Use of intravenous route for rapid medication administration:
   - Upsets the fine balance of homeostasis manifested in hives, acute urticaria, agitation, increased confusion, slurred speech

From Swonger, A., & Burbank, P. (1995). *Drug therapy and the elderly.* Boston: Jones and Bartlett Publishers, Inc.

- Introduce yourself (the nurse), by name.
- Tell me the date.
- What is the name of your street?
- Your phone number?
- Your birthday?
- How old are you?
- What would you do if your house caught on fire?
- In your mind, start with 100 and count back, subtracting by 7s
- Do you remember my name?

Table 13-6 is a commonly used tool to screen for depression; Table 13-7 measures cognition.

Laboratory Tests

Physiological processes and pathologies influence behavior and can mimic mental illness. The laboratory tests shown in Table 13-8 should be examined closely for high or high-normal results as well as low and low-normal results.

Table 13-6   Geriatric Depression Scale

THE GERIATRIC DEPRESSION SCALE (GDS)
By: Lenore Kurlowicz, PhD, RN, CS

WHY: Depression is common in late life, effecting nearly five million of the 31 million Americans aged 65 and older. Both major and minor depression are reproted in 13% of community dwelling older adults, 24% of older medical outpatients and 43% of both acute care and nursing home dwelling older adults. Contrary to popular belief, dpression is not a natural part of aging. Depression is often reversible with prompt and appropriate treatment. However, if left untreated, depression may result in the onset of physical, cognitive and social impariment as well as delayed recovery from medical illness and surgery, increased health care utilization and suicide.

BEST TOOL: While there are many instruments available to measure depression, the Geriatric Depression Scale (GDS), first created by Yesavage et al., has been tested and used extensively with the older population. It is a brief questionnaire in which participants are asked to respond to the 30 questions by answering yes or no in reference to how they felt on the day of administration. Scores of 0–10 are considered normal, 11–20 indicate mild depression and 21–30 indicate severe depression.

TARGET POPULATION: The GDS may be used with healthy, medically ill and mild to moderately cognitively impaired older adults. It has been extensively used in community, acute and long-term care settings.

VALIDITY/RELIABILITY: The GDS was found to have a 92% sensitivity and an 89% spcificity when evaluated against diagnostic criteria. The validity and reliability of the tool have been supported through both clinical practice and research.

STRENGTHS AND LIMITATIONS: The GDS is not a substitute for a diagnostic interview by mental health professionals. It is a useful screening tool in the clinical setting to facilitate assessment of depression in older adults especially when baseline measurements are compared to subsequent scores.

MORE ON THE TOPIC:
Koenig, H. G. Meador, K. G., Cohen, J. J. Blazer D. G. (1988). Self-rated depression scales and screening for major depression in the older hospitalized patient with medical illness. *Journal of the American Geriatrics Society,* 699–706.

Kurlowicz, L. H., & NICHE Faculty (1997). Nursing stand or practice protocol: Depression in elderly patients. *Geriatric Nursing,* 18, 192–199.

NIH Consensus Development Panel. (1992). Diagnosis and treatment of depression in late life. *JAMA, 268,* 1018–1024.

Sheikh, R. L. & Yesavage, J. A. (1986). Geriatric Depression Scale (GDS) recent evidence and development of a shorter version. *Clinical Gerontologist,* 5, 165–173.

Yesavage, J. A., Brink, T. L., Lum, O. Huang, V., Adey, M., Leirer, V. O. (1983). Development and validation of a geriatric depression screening scale: A preliminary report. *Journal of Psychiatric Research,* 17, 37–49.

Table 13-6 *(continued)*

Patient _____ Examiner _____ Date _____

Directions to Patient: Please choose the best answer for how you have felt over the past week.
Directions to Examiner: Present questions VERBALLY. Circle answer given by patient. Do not show to patient.

1. Are you basically satisfied with your life?	yes	**no** (1)
2. Have you dropped many of your activities and interests?	**yes** (1)	no
3. Do you feel that your life is empty?	**yes** (1)	no
4. Do you often get bored?	**yes** (1)	no
5. Are you hopeful about the future?	yes	**no** (1)
6. Are you bothered by thoughts you can't get out of your head?	**yes** (1)	no
7. Are you in good spirits most of the time?	yes	**no** (1)
8. Are you afraid that something bad is going to happen to you?	**yes** (1)	no
9. Do you feel happy most of the time?	yes	**no** (1)
10. Do you often feel helpless?	**yes** (1)	no
11. Do you often get restless and fidgety?	**yes** (1)	no
12. Do you prefer to stay home at night, rather than go out and do things?	**yes** (1)	no
13. Do you frequently worry about the future?	**yes** (1)	no
14. Do you feel you have more problems with memory than most?	**yes** (1)	no
15. Do you think it is wonderful to be alive now?	yes	**no** (1)
16. Do you feel downhearted and blue?	**yes** (1)	no
17. Do you feel pretty worthless the way you are now?	**yes** (1)	no
18. Do you worry a lot about the past?	**yes** (1)	no
19. Do you find life very exciting?	yes	**no** (1)
20. Is it hard for you to get started on new projects?	**yes** (1)	no
21. Do you feel full of energy?	yes	**no** (1)
22. Do you feel that your situation is hopeless?	**yes** (1)	no
23. Do you think that most people are better off than you are?	**yes** (1)	no
24. Do you frequently get upset over little things?	**yes** (1)	no
25. Do you frequently feel like crying?	**yes** (1)	no
26. Do you have trouble concentrating?	**yes** (1)	no
27. Do you enjoy getting up in the morning?	yes	**no** (1)
28. Do you prefer to avoid social occasions?	**yes** (1)	no
29. Is it easy for you to make decisions?	yes	**no** (1)
30. Is your mind as clear as it used to be?	yes	**no** (1)

TOTAL: Please sum all bolded answers (worth one point) for a total score. _____
Scores: 0–10 Normal   11–20 Moderate Depression   21–30 Severe Depression

Permission granted by **The Hartford Institute for Geriatric Nursing, Division of Nursing, New York University.** Available on the internet at www.nyu.edu/education/nursing/hartford.Institute.

Table 13-7   Mini-Mental State Exam (MMSE)

Score

_____

ORIENTATION
5   ____What is the (year), (season), (date), (day), (month)?
5   ____ Where are we: (state), (county), (town), (hospital), (floor).

REGISTRATION
3   ____ Name 3 objects: 1 second to say each. Then ask the patient all
             3 after you have said them. Give 1 point for each correct an-
             swer. Then repeat them until he learns all 3. Count number of
             trials and record.
Trials_____

ATTENTION AND CALCULATION
5   ___ Serial 7's. 1 point for each correct. Stop after 5 answers.Alterna-
             tively spell "world" backwards.

RECALL
3   ____ Ask for the 3 objects repeated above. Give 1 point for each
             correct.

LANGUAGE
9   ____ Name a pencil, and watch (**2** points). Repeat the following,
             "No ifs, ands or buts" (**1** point).
             Follow a three-stage command: "Take a paper in your right
             hand, fold it in half, and put it on the floor" (**3** points).
             Read and obey the following: "Close you eyes" (**1** point).
             Copy a design (**1** point) [2 intersecting pentagons]

TOTAL SCORE_____
Assess level of consciousness along a continuum:
             Alert   drowsy   stupor-coma

Instructions for administration of Mini-Mental State Exam

Orientation: 1. Ask for the date. Then ask specifically for parts omited,
e.g., "Can you also tell me what season it is?" One point for each correct
answer.
2. Ask in turn : "Can you tell me the name of this hospital?" (Town, county,
etc.). One point for each correct answer.
Registration: Ask the client if you may test his or her memory. Then say
the names of three unrelated objects, clearly and slowly, allowing about
one second for each. After you have said all three, ask him or her to repeat
them. This first repetition determines his or her score (0-3) but keep saying
them until he or she can repeat all three, up to 6 trials. If he or she does
not eventually learn all three, recall cannot be meaningfully tested.
Attention and Calculation: Ask the patient to begin with 100 and count
backwards by 7. Stop after 5 subtractions (93, 86, 79, 72, 65). Score the total
number of correct answers.

continued

Table 13-7   (continued)

If the patient cannot or will not perform this task, ask him or her to spell the word, "world" backwards. The score is the number of letters in correct order, e.g., dlrow = 5, dlorw = 3.

Recall: Ask the patient if he or she can recall the three words you previously asked him or her to remember. Score 0-3.

Language: *Naming*: Show the patient a wrist watch and ask him or her what it is. Repeat for pencil. Score 0-2.

Repetition: Ask the patient to repeat the sentence after you. Allow only one trial. Score 0 or 1.

Three-stage command: Give the patient a piece of plain blank paper and repeat the command. Score 1 point for each part correctly executed.

[A score of 21 or less out of a total of 30 possible points indicates possibility of cognitive impairment; further neurologiclaly assessment is warranted.]

From Folstein M., Folstein, S. & McHugh, P. (1975). Mini-mental state: A practical method for grading the cognitive state of patients for the clinician. *Journal of Psychiatric Research, 12,* 189–198. Copyright © 1975, 1998 MiniMental LLC.

Table 13-8   Laboratory Test Results—High or Low Levels May Affect Mental Status

- Standard blood chemistry profile
- Glucose FBS
- Thyroid function tests (T3,T4, TSH)
- Chest x-ray
- Urinalysis
- Electrocardiogram
- Digoxin, theophylline, psychotropic and benzodiazepine levels, if on these medications
- Syphilis test
- B12
- Folate/folic acid levels

Adapted from Simon Staab, A., & Compton Hodges, L. (1996). *Essentials of gerontological nursing: Adaptation to the aging process.* Philadelphia: Lippincott Company.

Depression, Delirium, and Dementia

Depression, delirium, and **dementia** are not normal aspects of aging. When and if any of the three syndromes occurs, it is important for the nurse to be able to distinguish them because treatment for each is very different. This is not an easy task, especially if an older adult already has underlying mental illness, depression, or dementia. Table 13-9 compares characteristics of the three syndromes.

Delirium is an acute episode of confusion often due to medication toxicity, infection, or pain in the older adult. Unlike dementia, where symptom control is realistic, delirium and depression are treatable and curable once the cause is uncovered. Antidepressant medication and psychotherapy can control depression. Similarly, treatment of medication toxicity, infection, and pain obliterate delirium, if treated immediately.

There are several types of dementia, each clinically presenting differently. Types of dementia include Alzheimer's dementia, vascular dementia, Creutzfeldt-Jakob disease, HIV-associated dementia, Huntington's disease, Parkinson's-associated dementia, and dementia associated with syphilis. The common elements of dementia include:

- The three "A"s: aphasia, apraxia, and agnosia
- Cognitive dysfunction

Table 13-9   Differentiating Delirium, Dementia, and Depression

Delirium	Dementia	Depression
• Acute, rapid onset: physiological disorder	• Gradual and progressive onset; organic disorder	• Rapid or gradual; affective disorder
• Reversible	• Irreversible	• Reversible
• Causes: medication toxicity, blood loss, infection, digoxin toxicity, pain, malnutrition, fluid and electrolyte imbalance	• Cause is unknown: organic in nature, mini strokes, viral	Cause: physiochemical and situational
• Pervades all activities	• Pervades all activities	• Pervades all activities
• Change in level of consciousness: hyper-awareness, hyper-activity	• No changes in level of consciousness	• Lethargic: diminished response to environmental stimuli
• Hallucinations/delusions present: seeing/hearing voices and others who are not there	• Affects cerebral cortex and sub-cortical structures: progressive retreat from reality	• Progressive distortion of reality: overwhelming sadness, lack of zest and pleasure for life
• Cannot concentrate long enough to answer questions asked; flight of thoughts	• Individual sincerely tries to answer questions asked	• Answers "don't know" to questions asked; implies "don't' care"
• Speaks in incomplete sentences	• Aphasia, apraxia, agnosia	• Coherent, slower speech

Content adapted from Matteson, M., McConnell, E., & Linton, A. (1997). *Gerontological nursing: Concepts and practice.* Philadelphia: W. B. Saunders Company.

• Memory loss
• Overall neurological decline

The treatment goals for dementia are provision of basic physiological needs, maintaining cognitive functioning for as long as possible, preservation of dignity, and advocacy for quality of life. Management of wandering and aggressive and paranoid behaviors, which may accompany dementia, presents major challenges to medical and nursing professionals. Some general guidelines are identified in Table 13-10.

NURSING TIPS

The most common presentation of tardive dyskinesia in an older person is tongue-thrusting, involuntary tongue movements, and facial movement (Jewell & Chemij, 1983; Masand, 2000). Make sure to rule out dental problems first.

Tardive Dyskinesia

Tardive dyskinesia (TD) is an iatrogenic (man-made) disorder; the discovery and use of **psychotropics** "created" this sec-

Table 13-10   Working with Behaviors Associated with Dementia

- Assess and understand wandering behavior:
  - When does the person wander?
  - Where does the person wander?
  - Is there a pattern to the wandering?
  - Is the wandering meaningful? Aimless? Frantic?
  - Is the individual looking for something? Hiding/running from something?
  - Are others present when wandering occurs?
  - What is the degree of environmental stimuli when the person is wandering?

- *Do not use physical restraints* if at all possible because they increase agitation and fear, are dehumanizing, and *do not promote safety.* They contribute to immobility, constipation, pressure ulcers, and decline in cognition.
- Aim "control" at the environment not at the individual. Create an environment, that is 'wanderer-friendly,' with lounges, places to rest and socialize, nontoxic plants, appropriate lighting, and personally meaningful items. Hospitals and homes present difficult challenges in this area:
  - Specialized medical and surgical hospital units for older adults with dementia is an ideal solution to working *with* instead of *against* the acute needs of this group.
  - Home care nurses working with family members recommend home safety strategies so that the older adult can safely wander throughout his or her own home, night or day.
  - Specially trained volunteers and appropriate adult care centers throughout the community provide companionship, activities, and care, again fitting the environment and stimuli to the person, not fitting the person to the environment.

- Try not to take aggressive behavior and angry statements personally. This is very difficult for nurses and others who have established long-standing relationships with an older adult with dementia. Seek out support groups and collegial support.
- Remain calm. Use a team approach that is nonviolent to help diffuse aggressive behaviors. Use pharmacological solutions as a last resort.
- Use gentle touch; do not rush the individual. Allow time for the older adult with dementia to acclimate to a new environment.
- Provide consistent caregivers when at all possible.
- Listen beyond what the person's words are saying; "listen" to feelings.
- Assure privacy, especially for those who exhibit socially inappropriate behaviors.
- Reflect on whether reality orientation is meaningful; validation therapy may be more suitable

ondary disease syndrome, which was recognized in the mid-1970s (Jewell & Chemij, 1983; Beeber, 1988). The exact cause of TD is not known. Theoretically, agitation at the dopamine receptors of the brain may be the culprit. TD is associated with long-term psychotropic usage (Masand, 2000). The symptoms include abnormal involuntary movements:

- head-nodding
- tongue-thrusting
- lip-smacking (most frequent symptom seen in older adults with this disorder)
- puckering, chewing, or sucking motions
- lateral jaw movements
- quick and jerky or slow, twisting movements in the trunk and upper and lower limbs

When the nurse identifies the presence of these symptoms, further neurological testing should be recommended. This condition is not necessarily reversible, but may be treated by prescribing drugs that block cholinergic receptors, withdrawing the psychotropic medication, or increasing the dose. Currently, a trial-and-error approach is practiced.

Strategies for Preserving Mental Health

Just as the body flourishes with moderate exercise and good nutrition, it also benefits from mental exercise and life-enhancing activities. These activities will vary person to person, given individual likes and dislikes within various cultures. Nevertheless, some basic principles follow. Dance, music, movement, pet therapy, and visits to child day care centers connect individuals to their environment and other people, and prove to be positive experiences. Similarly, group prayer and religious activities offer the hope and sense of strength needed to combat illness, loneliness, and depression, present in some older adults. A sharing of one's life experiences through a series of life review sessions (individual or group) is another way to help the older adult share his or her legacy with others. Mind games such as crossword puzzles or word and number games along with current event discus-

sions are cognitive exercises that keep the cerebral cortex functioning efficiently. Some routine in life tends to give structure and meaning to each day. Whether an older adult is at home, in a nursing home, or in the hospital, structure with degrees of flexibility should be established. Sense of reality and purpose goes along with such structure. For older adults who are no longer in touch with reality because of dementia, the nurse is able to validate and work within their reality in order to bring forth and reinforce the satisfaction with relationships and roles, which the older adult once felt in the past.

References

Beeber, L. (1988). It's on the tip of the tongue; Tardive dyskinesia. *Journal of Psychosocial Nursing, 26*, 8.

Burke, M., & Walsh, M. (1997). *Gerontologic nursing: Wholistic care of the older adult* (2nd ed.). St. Louis: Mosby-Year Book, Inc.

Estes, M. E. Z. (1998). *Health assessment and physical examination.* Albany: Delmar Thomson Learning.

Folstein, M., Folstein, S., & McHugh, P. (1975). Mini-mental state: A practical method for grading the cognitive state of patients for the clinician. *Journal of Psychiatric Research, 12*, 189–198.

Frisch, N., & Frisch, L. (1998). *Psychiatric mental health nursing.* Albany: Delmar Publishers.

Jewell, J., & Chemij, M. (1983). Tardive dyskinesia: The involuntary movement disorder that no one really understands. *Canadian Nurse, 79*, 20–24.

Masand, P. S. (2000). Side effects of antipsychotics in the elderly. *J of Clinical Psychiatry, 61*, Supp18, 43–49.

Matteson, M., McConnell, E., & Linton, A. (1997). *Gerontological nursing: Concepts and practice* (2nd ed.). Chapter 15. Philadelphia: W. B. Saunders Co.

Simon Staab, A., & Compton Hodges, L. (1996). *Essentials of gerontological nursing: Adaptation to the aging process.* Philadelphia: J. B. Lippincott Company.

Swonger, A., & Burbank, P. (1995). *Drug therapy and the elderly.* Boston: Jones and Bartlett Publishers.

Yesavage, J. & Brink, T. (1983). Development and validation of a geriatric depression screening scale: A preliminary report. *Journal of Psychiatric Research, 17,* 37–49.

14

Nutritional Assessment

Key Terms

anorexia
cachexia
dehydration
failure to thrive (FTT)
Food Guide Pyramid
Malnutrition
Nutrition Screening Initiative (NSI)
registered dietician (R.D.)
Recommended dietary allowances (RDAs)

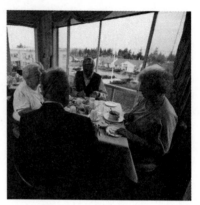

The nutritional assessment of an older adult should be conducted in conjunction with a **registered dietician** in the nursing home, home care, or hospital setting. It is based on an understanding of risk factors associated with nutritional status. The assessment includes subjective data on the food preferences of the individual along with objective data on psychosocial variables, patterns in weight gain/losses, food habits established over the years, and medication interaction. In addition, socioeconomic as well as the cultural context within the person's lifestyle are examined in order to identify nutritional problems such as **malnutrition,** inadequate hydration, **anorexia,** overeating, or muscle wasting **(cachexia).** Analysis of results from selective laboratory tests contributes to the overall assessment of nutritional status of the older adult.

Risk Factors

Multiple factors contribute to substandard nutritional levels in the older adult. They include:

- Acute or chronic illness
- Poor dentition
- Immobility
- Dysphagia
- History of bone pain
- Dependency/disability
- Neglect and abuse, physical or mental
- Advanced age (> 80)
- Poor appetite
- Low calcium intake
- Poverty
- Social isolation
- Chronic medication use

(This list was adapted from the Nutritional Screening Initiative [1992], a joint program of the American Academy of Family Physicians, the National Council on Aging and the American Dietetic Association.)

Many older adults exhibit at least two or more of these factors, placing them at risk for lowered nutritional levels. Hence, interview questions and health assessment observations surround screening and identification of these risk factors.

Normal Age-Related Nutritional Changes and Psychosocial Factors

Tables 14-1 and 14-2 include a summary of age-related changes affecting nutritional status, and psychosocial factors, respectively. Most of the age-related factors cannot be directly controlled, although medical nutritionists say that vitamin and mineral supplementation is beneficial.

Table 14-1   Age-Related Changes in Older Adults That Affect Nutritional Status

Decreases in:
- Metabolism with concurrent decreased need in total caloric intake
- Muscle mass, with increase in fatty tissue
- Peristalsis and movement of food through the gastrointestinal tract
- Hydrochloric acid and saliva
- Taste buds and olfactory efficiency
- Teeth (increased tooth loss and periodontal disease)
- Visual acuity, as it affects food ingestion and preparation
- Mild decrease in swallowing ability
- Increases in medication usage, which often reduce nutrient absorption

Summarized from Burke, M., & Walsh, M. (1997). Gerontologic nursing: *Wholistic care of the older adult.* St. Louis: Mosby-Year Book, Inc.;

Matteson, M., McConnell, E. S., & Linton, A. (1997). *Gerontological nursing: Concepts and practice.* Philadelphia: W. B. Saunders Company

Table 14-2   Psychosocial Factors Affecting Older Adults' Nutritional Status

- Low income
- Loneliness
- Depression
- Social isolation
- Substance abuse
- Sensory losses
- Hopelessness

- Six to eleven servings from bread, cereal, rice, and pasta groups
- Three to five servings from the vegetable group
- Two to four servings from the fruit group
- Two to three servings from the milk, yogurt, and cheese group
- Two to three servings from the meat, poultry, fish, dry beans, eggs, and nuts group
- Fats, oils, and sweets in small amounts

The Food Guide Pyramid

The Food Guide Pyramid (Figure 14-1), published by the U.S. Department of Agriculture and Health and Human Services (1992), offers basic guidelines for portions and food selection. It encourages daily servings of the following:

The Food Guide Pyramid is considered a safe guideline for older adults. Caloric intake may need to be adjusted if the older adult is underweight or overweight.

RDAs are "recommended dietary allowances of nutrients". Although RDAs are known for adults, they are not specific to *older* adults. Therefore, under RDA guidelines, it appears as though the RDAs of a

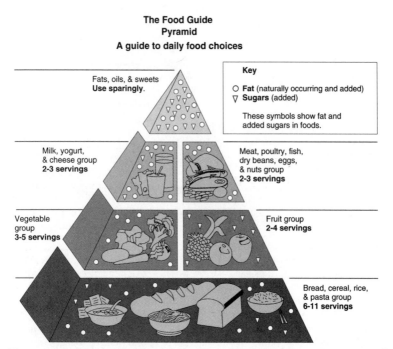

The Food Guide Pyramid
A guide to daily food choices

Key
○ **Fat** (naturally occurring and added)
▽ **Sugars** (added)

These symbols show fat and added sugars in foods.

Fats, oils, & sweets
Use sparingly.

Milk, yogurt, & cheese group
2-3 servings

Meat, poultry, fish, dry beans, eggs, & nuts group
2-3 servings

Vegetable group
3-5 servings

Fruit group
2-4 servings

Bread, cereal, rice, & pasta group
6-11 servings

Figure 14-1   Food Guide Pyramid. Courtesy of the United States Department of Agriculture and the United States Department of Health and Human Services (1992).

55-year-old are the same as those for a 90-year-old. Nutritionists and other health care practitioners feel that nutritional needs differ in the young-old and old-old. Again, the Food Guide Pyramid is probably one of the best guidelines for balanced nutrition for older adults. Currently, vitamin and mineral supplementation is gaining recognition and support in the scientific community. Additional vitamin C, zinc, and coenzyme Q10 are some examples of accepted supplementation.

Nutritional Assessment Tools and Significant Findings

Through interaction and health history taking of the older adult and, if appropriate, significant family members, baseline data is obtained from which to plan care. Nutritional screening includes a set of open-ended yet specific questions, a 24-hour dietary history, height, weight, and brief family history. Although the nurse is usually not in a position to obtain anthropometric measurements that determine body fat, the registered dietician (RD) may have the equipment for triceps skinfold measurement (TSF), midarm circumference (MAC), and midarm muscle circumference (MAMC), or the results of these tests may be available. Tables 14-3, 14-4, and 14-5 depict the nutritional history, assessment, significant physical assessment findings, and lab data.

Alcohol, tobacco use, and illegal substances effect nutritional status. Establish rapport and trust with the older adult. Ensure that you, the nurse, are not there to "pass judgment" on behaviors. Be sensitive to self-neglect, which may manifest itself as anorexia, obesity, and/or disheveled appearance.

Severe depression and hopelessness may be underlying causes of self-inflicted starvation. In this case, the nurse should branch off into questions such as, "You seem sad. Would you like to talk about what is bothering you?" If the older adult says, "I hate the nursing home," or "I hate living at home," use the technique of mirroring ("You hate living at home [in the nursing home]?"). This therapeutic response assists the nurse in getting at the heart of a seemingly nutritional issue.

Findings of protein calorie malnutrition especially in the nursing home, are not an uncommon problem. The manner in which residents are being fed and the types of food being served, presence and progression of underlying diseases such as diabetes, endocrine disorders, and renal disease, as well as competence of CNAs must be scrutinized. "Spot checking" at mealtime and role modeling through assisting with feeding residents will help to ensure that quality is not being sacrificed for speed.

Weight loss is a foreboding sign in older adults who are not trying to reduce weight. If the nurse's findings include weight loss of 5 to 10 pounds per year or 5 pounds per month in a nursing home, other investigation or questioning regarding family history of cancer or the client's history of cancer, thyroid/endocrine or other chronic illness should be pursued.

NURSING TIPS

Weighing an older adult is deceptive. In order to be accurate, weights must be taken at the same time of day, wearing the same clothing. Consistency is the key to accurate weights. If three individuals are weighing a person, the odds of the *exact same* methods being used are somewhat unlikely. In some instances, medication adjustments are made based on a weight (e.g., diuretic dosages). The nurse has the responsibility to instruct and inform staff of the importance of consistency in protocol on taking weights.

Last but certainly not of least importance is the influence of religion and culture on food choices. For many older adults, food habits are connected to traditions that transmigrated from their mother countries—(Spain, Italy, China, Korea, Africa, etc.). The meaning of the traditions and

Table 14-3   Nutritional Screening

HISTORY

In the past 6–12 months:

- Have you experienced any change in weight?
- Has your appetite or dietary habits changed?
- Do you have any difficulty in feeding self, eating, chewing, or swallowing?
- Have you experienced any nausea, vomiting, or diarrhea?
- What are your food likes and dislikes?
- How do you prepare and store your food?
- Do you eat alone or with a family or group?
- Do you take any vitamins or supplements (liquid diets)?
- Do you follow a particular diet?
- Do you have any especially strong cravings.

Review 24-hour diet history:

Time Food Eaten	Amount	Method of Preparation	Where Eaten

ASSESSMENT

Appearance of Patient

Height _____ feet & inches/cm
Weight _____ lb/kg

- Do you have any familial risk factors, such as obesity, high cholesterol, diabetes mellitus, hypertension, coronary artery disease, cerebrovascular disease, or cancer?
- What nutritional concerns would you like to discuss?

associated foods or fasting must be analyzed related to the health of the older adult. Fasting, in some cultures, is part of religious holidays and cultural events. Most religions make exceptions for the very young or very old in recognition of their sensitivity and need for food and fluids. If necessary, the nurse may want to speak with the rabbi or priest to gain respect and perspective on the norms and choices older adults may adhere to during religious holidays. Also, it is wise not to pass judgment on foods that older adults indulge in during religious or sectarian holidays. Generally, high-fat, high-salt, and high-sugar foods *in moderation* two

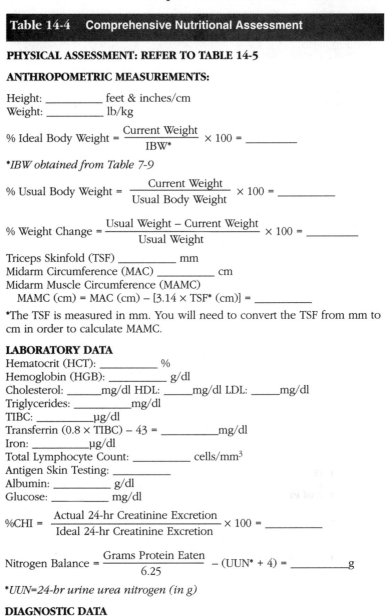

Table 14-4 Comprehensive Nutritional Assessment

PHYSICAL ASSESSMENT: REFER TO TABLE 14-5

ANTHROPOMETRIC MEASUREMENTS:

Height: _____ feet & inches/cm
Weight: _____ lb/kg

$$\% \text{ Ideal Body Weight} = \frac{\text{Current Weight}}{\text{IBW}^*} \times 100 = \underline{\hspace{1cm}}$$

IBW obtained from Table 7-9

$$\% \text{ Usual Body Weight} = \frac{\text{Current Weight}}{\text{Usual Body Weight}} \times 100 = \underline{\hspace{1cm}}$$

$$\% \text{ Weight Change} = \frac{\text{Usual Weight} - \text{Current Weight}}{\text{Usual Weight}} \times 100 = \underline{\hspace{1cm}}$$

Triceps Skinfold (TSF) _____ mm
Midarm Circumference (MAC) _____ cm
Midarm Muscle Circumference (MAMC)
  MAMC (cm) = MAC (cm) – [3.14 × TSF* (cm)] = _____

*The TSF is measured in mm. You will need to convert the TSF from mm to cm in order to calculate MAMC.

LABORATORY DATA

Hematocrit (HCT): _____ %
Hemoglobin (HGB): _____ g/dl
Cholesterol: _____mg/dl HDL: _____mg/dl LDL: _____mg/dl
Triglycerides: _____mg/dl
TIBC: _____µg/dl
Transferrin (0.8 × TIBC) – 43 = _____mg/dl
Iron: _____µg/dl
Total Lymphocyte Count: _____ cells/mm^3
Antigen Skin Testing: _____
Albumin: _____ g/dl
Glucose: _____ mg/dl

$$\%\text{CHI} = \frac{\text{Actual 24-hr Creatinine Excretion}}{\text{Ideal 24-hr Creatinine Excretion}} \times 100 = \underline{\hspace{1cm}}$$

$$\text{Nitrogen Balance} = \frac{\text{Grams Protein Eaten}}{6.25} - (\text{UUN}^* + 4) = \underline{\hspace{1cm}} \text{g}$$

UUN=24-hr urine urea nitrogen (in g)

DIAGNOSTIC DATA
X-rays _____

or three times per year hold sociocultural, psychosocial, and religious benefits superceding the physiological risks.

Nursing diagnoses related to nutritional issues are shown in Table 14-6.

Hydration Issues

It is hypothesized that most older adults do not drink 1000 cc of fluid daily. In fact, the fluids they ingest comprise liquids that

Table 14-5   Physical Signs and Symptoms of Poor Nutritional Status

	Subjective	Objective
1. General appearance	Fatigue, poor sleep, change in weight, frequent infections	Dull affect, apathetic, increased weight, decreased weight
2. Skin	Pruritus, swelling, delayed wound healing	Dry, rough, scaling, flaky, edema, lesions, decreased turgor, changes in color (pallor, jaundice), petechiae, ecchymoses, xanthomas (slightly elevated yellow nodules)
3. Nails	Brittle	Dry, splinter hemorrhages, spoon-shaped, pale
4. Hair	Easily falls out, brittle	Less shiny, dry, changes in color pigment
5. Eyes	Vision changes, night blindness, eye discharge	Hardening and scaling of cornea, conjunctiva pale or red
6. Mouth	Mouth sores	Lips: cracked, dry, swollen, fissures around corners Gums: recessed, swollen, bleeding, spongy Tongue: smooth, beefy red, magenta, pale, fissures, sores, increased or decreased in size, increased or decreased papillae Teeth: missing, caries
7. Head and neck	Headaches, decreased hearing	Xanthelasma, irritation and crusting of nares, swollen cheeks (parotid gland enlargement), goiter
8. Heart and peripheral vasculature	Palpitations, swelling	Cardiac enlargement, changes in blood pressure, tachycardia, heart murmur, edema
9. Abdomen	Tender, changes in appetite, nausea, changes in bowel habits	Edema, hepatosplenomegaly
10. Musculoskeletal system	Weakness, pain, cramping, frequent fractures	Muscle tone is decreased, flabby muscles, bowing of lower extremities
11. Neurological system	Irritable, changes in mood, numbness, paresthesia	Slurred speech, unsteady gait, tremors, decreased deep tendon reflexes, loss of position and vibratory sense, paresthesia, decreased coordination

Table 14-6   Some Sample Nutrition-Related Nursing Diagnoses

- Alteration in nutrition, less than or greater than body requirement
- Alteration in body image
- Impaired swallowing
- Fluid volume deficit, related to decrease in fluid intake

have a diuretic effect, such as coffee, tea, and high-sugar juices (Zembrzuski, 1997). If the nurse suspects subclinical **dehydration** in an older adult, the assessment tool in Table 14-7 could be used for more comprehensive and in-depth data. Water is a vital portion (60 to 70 percent) of body composition and should be treated seriously. See Table 14-8 for a summary of dehydration findings in older adults.

Laboratory Data

Decreased or increased blood levels of specific substances in the body are reflective of nutritional problems, within the context of the health history and exam findings. Table 14-9 lists lab levels, which should be examined carefully for borderline or above-/below-normal results. Remember that older adults may be symptomatic when levels read normal. On the other hand, they may show *no symptoms* when lab levels are *not normal.* Lab levels alone are not a reliable indicator of illness; they must be analyzed in light of the clinical picture.

Failure to Thrive Syndrome

Failure to thrive syndrome (FTT) in older adults is a relatively new concept (Braun, Wycle, & Cowling, 1988). It manifests itself as unexplained weight loss and malnutrition (Newbern, 1992). Usually, these older adults have complex, numerous problems, and lose their will to live. Although there is research on failure to

thrive and attachment behavior in infants, little information exists on the syndrome in older adults. It is thought that the ability to bond and connect with society falls apart in some older adults. As this occurs, the person becomes overwhelmed and despondent, resulting in a giving up on self and others.

What can the nurse do if FTT is suspected? An in-depth social history as well as a nutritional and mental status assessment is paramount to formulating nursing diagnoses and interventions. With proper nutrition, psychiatric interventions, reminiscence therapy, and pharmacological treatment, FTT can be turned around.

References

Braun, J., Wycle, M., & Cowling, W. (1988). Failure to thrive in older persons: A concept derived. *Gerontologist, 28,* 809–812.

Burke, M., & Walsh, M. (1997) *Gerontologic nursing: Wholistic care of the older adult.* St. Louis: Mosby-Year Book, Inc.

Estes, M. E. Z (1998). *Health assessment and physical examination.* Albany: Delmar Publishers.

Matteson, M., McConnell, E. S., & Linton, A. (1997). *Gerontological nursing: Concepts and practice.* Chapter 19. Philadelphia: W. B. Saunders Company.

Newbern, V. (1992). Failure to thrive: A growing concern in the elderly. *Journal of gerontological nursing,* 21–25.

Nutritional Screening Initiative. (1997). Determine your nutritional health. A project of the American Academy of Family Physicians, the American Dietetic Association, and the National Council on the Aging, Inc., and funded in part by a grant from Ross Products Division, Abbott Laboratories. Washington, DC.

Quinn, C. (1997). *The Nutritional Screening Initiative: Meeting the nutritional needs of elders. Orthopedic Nursing,* 16(6), 13–24.

Zembrzuski, C. D. (1999). Failure to thrive,

Table 14-7   Comprehensive Nursing Assessment Checklist to Identify Residents at High Risk for Decreased Fluid Intake

Purpose: to promote hydration, prevent dehydration
Name of resident:_____   Name of nurse: _____
Unit:
Date:

Check off those assessment findings characteristic of the resident. The greater the number of factors or severity of factors, the greater the risk for diminished hydration. Add descriptive clinical comments as needed.
I. Symptoms of dehydration warranting immediate medical and nursing interventions:

___ Fever
___ Thirst (not a reliable indicator in elders)
___ Dry, warm skin
___ Dry mucous membranes
___ More than one lengthwise division of the tongue (furrowed)
___ Decreased urinary output
___ Concentrated urine
___ Muscular weakness
___ Diminished skin turgor *less than usual baseline* (test over sternum or forehead)
___ Increased lethargy
___ Daily weight loss
___ Increased confusion, greater than usual
___ Change in baseline mental function
___ Constipation
___ Sunken eyes (severe dehydration)
___ Tachycardia (severe dehydration)
___ Hypotension (severe dehydration)

II. Factors associated with hydration problems:
___ Age 85 or older
___ Physical immobility (cannot get to water, cannot hold cup: assess functional status)
___ Current dysphagia; mechanical problems in swallowing
___ Cognitive impairment
    A. Unable to request fluids
    B. Unaware of thirst
___ Incontinent of urine
___ Fluid intake of 1500 ml or less (do not include caffeinated drinks)
    Attach 2 to 3 days of intake and output:
        A. Day 1
        B. Day 2
        C. Day 3
___ Documented impaired oral intake over the past 1 to 2 weeks:
    Estimated date of onset:
___ Currently on intake and output monitoring
___ Resident spends most of the day outdoors in dry and hot temperatures 80°F or warmer

Table 14-7 (continued)

___ Resident is active or exercises for at least 30 minutes daily or every other day
III. Problems increasing vulnerability
   A. Medical
      ___ Hypertension
      ___ Kidney disease
      ___ Congestive heart failure
      ___ Any type of dementia
      ___ Central nervous system disorders
      ___ Osteoarthritis
      ___ Osteoporosis
      ___ Uncontrolled diabetes
   B. Dietary restrictions
      ___ Fluids
      ___ Salt
      ___ Potassium
      ___ Protein
   C. Medications
      ___ Diuretics   List:
      ___ Tricyclic antidepressants or lithium   List:
      ___ Regular use of laxatives   List:
   D. Medical history
      ___ Dehydration
      ___ Fever
      ___ Diarrhea/vomiting
      ___ Infections
      ___ Difficulty swallowing
   E. Immediate return from
      ___ One day or greater hospitalization
      ___ Diagnostic testing requiring use of contrast dyes
      ___ Dental surgery
      ___ Eye surgery
      ___ One-day clinic visit
      ___ Any test requiring administration of nothing by mouth after midnight
IV. Laboratory reports showing *steady increases** in
___ Sodium
___ Serum blood urea nitrogen
___ Creatinine
___ Hematocrit
___ Serum osmolality
___ Urine specific gravity

*Look *for upward changes* in these baseline laboratory values over time; unless the resident is severely dehydrated, these laboratory values may remain within normal limits but will climb slowly as hydration deteriorates

Nurse's signature:

Other pertinent clinical comments by the nurse and the interdisciplinary team followed by signatures:

Table 14-8   Summary on Dehydration Findings

- Hypernatremia (high blood sodium)
- Decrease in total body water
- Increased blood urea nitrogen (BUN)
- Increased creatinine
- Increased hematocrit
- Increased serum osmolality
- Concentrated urine (increased urine specific gravity)
- Minimal urinary output
- Confusion and change in mental status
- Sunken eyes, in later stages
- Dry, warm skin; furrowed tongue; fever, in later stages
- Tachycardia and weak thready pulse, in later stages
- Orthostatic hypotension

Adapted from Zembrzuski, C. (1997). A three-dimensional approach to hydration of elders: Administration, clinical staff, and in-service education, *Geriatric Nursing, 18*(1), 24–25.

depression and dehydration: Related concepts. Unpublished paper: New York University.

Zembrzuski, C. D. (1997). A three-dimensional approach to hydration of elders: Administration, clinical staff, and in-service education. *Geriatric Nursing, 18*(1), 24–29.

Table 14-9   Laboratory Test Findings Potentially Supporting Impaired Nutrition

- Hemoglobin: < 12.0g/dl; hematocrit < 35
- Serum albumin: < 3.5g/dl
- Total lymphocyte count: < 800 cells/mms (severe protein deficiency)
- Fasting glucose: < 70 and > 110 mg/dl
- Cholesterol: < 140 or > 220
- Low-density lipoproteins (LDLs): > 160
- High-density lipoproteins (HDLs): > 85
- Triclycerides: > 150 or < 35
- Increased or decreased levels of transferrin: less than 170 or greater than 250 mg/dl (indicates anemia, iron-deficient state)
- Total iron binding capacity (TIBC): < 240 or > 450 micrograms/dl
- Serum iron (women): < 65 or > 165 micrograms/dl
- Serum iron (men): < 74 or > 175 micrograms/dl
- 24-hour urine for nitrogen: excessive nitrogen from tissue breakdown is abnormal
- Antigen skin testing test such as PPD tuberculin test or *Candida albicans* skin tests: delayed positive reaction due to low numbers of antibodies indicative of malnutrition
- Creatinine Height Index (CHI): based on a 24-hour urine, 80 to 90 percent indicates mild protein deficiency; 70 to 80 percent moderate; < 70 percent severe
- Bone density x-rays showing osteoporosis

Adapted from Estes, M. E. Z. (1998). *Health assessment and physical examination.* Albany: Delmar Publishers.

15

Abdominal Assessment

Key Terms

borborygmi
clicks and gurgles
colostomy
Crohn's disease
Cullen's sign
gastroesophogeal reflex disorder
   (GERD)
hemorrhoids
hepatic
hiatal hernia
ileostomy
irritable bowel disease
mononucleosis
peptic ulcer disease
peritoneum
tympany
urinary tract infections (UTIs)
venous hum

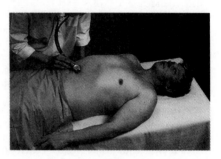

TIPS FROM THE EXPERTS

Complaint of "abdominal discomfort" must always be investigated. Abdominal discomfort affects appetite, contributes to weight loss, and detracts from socialization and
recreational activities. It may also be a warning sign of a
serious problem. Medication groups such as the nons-
teroidal anti-inflammatory drugs (NSAIDS) may cause internal bleeding. anti-hyperlipidemic drugs may produce
gas, bloating, and diarrhea.

An abdominal assessment in older adults is reflective of gastrointestinal, genitourinary, digestive, and **hepatic** (liver) health and functioning. Abdominal-related complaints are common in older adults. Thus, it is difficult to distinguish minor from major problems. The abdomen comprises the stomach, large and small intestines, kidneys, spleen, liver, gallbladder, pancreas, vermiform appendix, ureters, and bladder—virtually every organ between the diaphragm and symphysis pubis. A detailed, thorough abdominal assessment including client history, inspection, auscultation, percussion, and palpation, in that order, reveals necessary data warranting more aggressive nursing and diagnostic interventions. Figures 15-1 and 15-2 and Table 15-1 depict the structures, quadrants, and anatomic map of the abdomen requiring clinician familiarity.

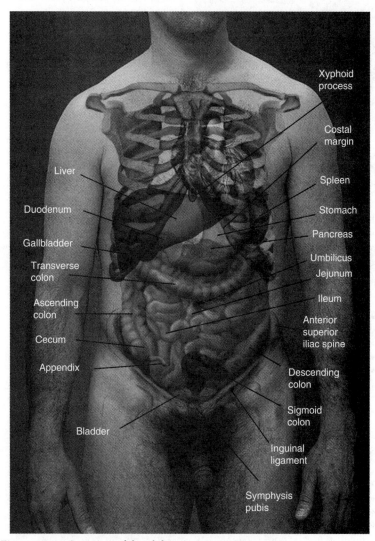

Figure 15-1   Structures of the Abdomen: Anterior View

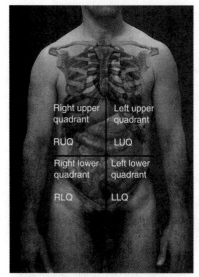

Figure 15-2   Abdominal Quadrants

Client History and Age-Related Changes in the Abdomen

The medical, surgical, and social history of the older adult should include relevant information as shown in Table 15-2.

Table 15-3 depicts age-related changes in the abdominal organs, based on current research and knowledge. Note that some changes are not conclusively related to advancing age.

Inspection

The nurse observes for contour of the abdomen, symmetry, muscle usage, pigmentation, scars, striae, respiratory movement, notable masses, pulsations, and shape of the umbilicus.

Contour of the abdomen, while the older adult is in the supine position, is flat or slightly rounded. A distended abdomen may indicate any of the following problems (known as the 7 "F"s):

- Fat
- Fluid (ascites)
- Flatus
- Feces (left-sided distension over quadrant may indicate impaction)
- Fatal growth (malignancy)
- Fibroid tumor
- [Fetus]

Asymmetry is an abnormal finding indicative of tumor, cyst, obstruction, or scolio-

Table 15-1   Four-Quadrant Anatomic Map

Right Upper Quadrant (RUQ)	Left Upper Quadrant (LUQ)
• Liver • Gallbladder • Pylorus • Duodenum • Pancreas (head) • Portion of right kidney and adrenal gland • Hepatic flexure of colon • Section of ascending and transverse colons	• Left lobe of liver • Stomach • Spleen • Pancreas (body) • Portion of left kidney and adrenal gland • Splenic flexure of colon • Sections of transverse and descending colons

Right Lower Quadrant (RLQ)	Left Lower Quadrant (LLQ)
• Appendix • Cecum • Lower pole of right kidney • Right ureter • Right ovary (female) • Right spermatic cord (male)	• Sigmoid colon • Section of descending colon • Lower pole of left kidney • Left ureter • Left ovary (female) • Left spermatic cord (male)

✓ **NURSING CHECKLIST**

General Approach to Abdominal Assessment

- Ensure that the room is at a warm, comfortable temperature to prevent client chilling and shivering.
- Utilize an adequate light source. This includes both a bright, overhead light and a freestanding lamp for tangential lighting.
- Ask the client to urinate before the examination.
- Drape the client from the xiphoid process to the symphysis pubis, then expose the client's abdomen.
- To ensure abdominal relaxation, position the client comfortably in a supine position with knees flexed over a pillow, or position the client so that the arms are either folded across the chest or at the sides.
- Have client point to tender areas: assess these last. Mark these and other significant findings (e.g., scars, dullness) on the body diagram in the client's chart.
- Watch the client's face closely for signs of discomfort or pain.

Table 15-2   Abdominal-Related Assessment Data to Obtain from the Older Adult

Medical, history of:
- Tumors
- **Peptic ulcer disease**
- **Gastroesophogeal reflux disorder (GERD)**
- Renal failure, chronic or acute
- Gallstones, kidney stones
- Infections: parasitic, food poisoning, **urinary tract (UTIs), mononucleosis**
- **Hemorrhoids**, rectal bleeding
- Pancreatitis, appendicitis, cholecystitis, colitis, hepatitis
- **Irritable bowel disease**, intestinal blockages
- **Crohn's disease**

Surgical, history of:
- Cholecystectomy, gastrectomy
- **Ileostomy, colostomy**
- Colectomy, nephrectomy, splenectomy
- **Hiatal hernia** repair
- Transplant: liver, renal

Social history:
- Altered nutrition
- Gastric absorption impairment
- Alcohol use
- Abuse/neglect

Adapted from Cauthorne-Burnette, T., & Estes, M. E. Z. (1998). *Clinical companion for health assessment and physical examination.* Albany: Delmar Publishers.

Table 15-3   Abdominal Changes Experienced by Some Older Adults

- Decreased esophageal motility usually due to neurological disease, *not* healthy aging
- Swallowing difficulties, *not* due to healthy aging
- Atrophy of gastric mucosa
- Decreased hydrochloric acid (hydrochlorhydria)
- Absorption in small intestines (debatable)
- Some decreased motility in large intestines
- *Constipation is *not* part of normal aging
  - decreased fiber and water and drug therapy affect bowel function
- Pancreatic changes, with mixed findings
  - Increase in pancreatic ducts, decrease in pancreatic weight
  - Increase calcification of pancreatic vessels
  - Bicarbonate, amylase, trypsin remain unchanged
- Decreased liver weight
  - Decrease in hepatic cells
- Decrease in cholesterol and bile acid synthesis
  - Decreased clearance of benzodiazepines

Adapted from Matteson, M., McConnell, E., & Linton, A. (1997). *Gerontological nursing: Concepts and practice.* Philadelphia: W. B. Saunders Company.

ments of the abdomen should be smooth and even; retractions are indicative of pathologies such as pancreatitis or perforated ulcer.

It is unusual but peristalsis movement may be observed in a lean older adult. These observable ripples moving down the abdomen may suggest intestinal obstruction. Pulsation of the abdominal aorta may be visible. If bounding, an aneurysm or right ventricular hypertrophy may be present. The umbilicus is indented beneath the abdominal surface. If protruding, an umbilical hernia, ascites, or carcinoma is suggested.

NURSING TIPS

The most common sources of abdominal scarring are appendectomy, hysterectomy, and cesarean section. On the body diagram in the client's chart, document the location, size, and condition of all scars.

NURSING TIPS

Constipation is a common problem in older people. In general, it is preventable. First, adequate fluid must be ingested. Second, the older person must commit to a diet high in fiber. Third, moderate exercise must be maintained for circulation and movement of lymphatic fluids. Before pharmacological interventions are prescribed, these three steps should be tried.

sis. If the client is able to raise the head and shoulders off the exam table, note the abdominal muscles. Inspect for scars and pigmentation. **Cullen's sign** (blue around umbilicus suggesting blood in peritoneal cavity), engorged abdominal veins suggesting circulatory problems, and scars indicating surgeries or injuries are documented.

Striae, masses, or nodules are abnormal findings and may indicate metastases or malignancies. Likewise, respiratory move-

Auscultation

Auscultation precedes palpation and percussion to prevent prompted exaggerated bowel sounds. Place the warmed diaphragm of the stethoscope on each quadrant: RLQ, RUQ, LUQ, and LLQ. Listen for 5 minutes at each quadrant. Per quadrant, 5 to 30 times per minute, of "clicks and gurgles" is considered normal. **Borborygmi** is the term used for hyperactive bowel sounds—loud, noisy, high-pitched sounds often audible without the use of the stethoscope. Abnormal findings include no sounds or sounds greater than 30/5 min./ quadrant, indicative of obstruction or gastroenteritis, respectively. A **venous hum** is also abnormal. This is a continuous vibratory low- to medium-pitched sound. If heard, cirrhosis of the liver is a potential pathology.

Auscultate for bruits by placing the bell of the stethoscope over the abdominal aorta, renal arteries, and femoral arteries. Placement is shown in Figure 15-3.

Bruits indicate stenosis or aortic aneurysm.

Friction rubs, which sound like pieces of sandpaper rubbing together, suggest inflammation of the **peritoneum,** possibly caused by a tumor or infarct. Friction rubs are best heard by placing the diaphragm of the stethoscope placed over right and left costal margins, liver, and spleen.

Percussion

Familiarity with the organs throughout each of the four quadrants is paramount to successful and effective percussion. The key to percussion is being able to listen and note when **tympany** progresses to dullness. Tympany is the norm because of air in the intestines and stomach. Dullness may suggest a tumor or full intestine. Table 15-4 reviews sounds related to abdominal assessment.

NURSING TIPS

Percussion sounds reflect different densities in the body. By placing the index or middle finger over a body location, then tapping that finger with the opposite middle finger, a sound is produced: flat, dull, resonant, hyper-resonant, or tympanic. It is helpful to know when the older adult last ate and had a bowel movement in interpreting assessment findings. More detail is offered in Chapter 2 on physical assessment techniques.

Percuss the liver by beginning at the right midclavicular line below the umbilicus up to the lower part of the liver (mark off). Sounds change from tympanic to dull.

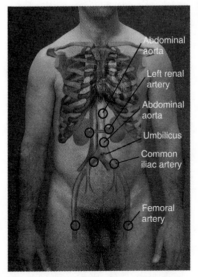

Figure 15-3 Stethoscope Placement for Ascultating Abdominal Vasculature

Table 15-4 Sounds Commonly Heard in the Abdomen

Borborygmi	loud gurgles; "noisy stomach"; may be heard without stethoscope; hyper-activity
Bruits	swishing sound
Venous hum	continual, vibrating noise
Friction rub	sounds like sand-paper rubbing together
Tympany	hollow, high-pitched long duration, like a drum implying emptiness
Dullness	high-pitched, moderate duration implying moderate density

Next, percuss downward from right mid-clavicular line to where lung resonance changes to dullness (mark off). Measure. Six to 12 centimeters is a normal finding for liver span, based on the size of the individual. Note that it may not always be possible to mark off liver span because of the older client's preference, fears, and mentation. Also, adipose tissue may make it difficult to accurately assess the liver.

Liver descent is measured by subtracting the difference between liver border upon inspiration and exhalation. During inhalation, percuss the lower border of the liver by noting tympany to dullness at the right midclavicular line (mark off). Do the same after exhalation. Mark off. A 2 to 3 centimeter difference is normal; greater than 2 to 3 centimeters suggests hepatomegaly. Less than 2 centimeters suggest tumor or ascites.

Percuss the spleen, which is located in the LUQ. Percuss posterior to the midaxillary line downward until dullness is heard (see Figure 15-4).

Six to 8 centimeters dullness between the left costal margin, from the sixth to the tenth rib, is a normal finding. Splenomegaly exists if dullness is beyond 8 centimeters above the left costal margin.

Percuss the stomach in the LUQ at left lower anterior rib cage and left epigastric area. Tympany, if the stomach is empty, is normal.

To check for kidney and liver tenderness, "fist percussion" is used. This type of percussion is important not to overlook because of the potential for polynephritis, hepatitis, and cholecystitis. Pain is never a normal response to physical examination. Direct and indirect fist percussion of the left kidney is shown in Figures 15-5A and 15-5B.

The fist is placed over the costovertebral angle (Figure 15-5A) and struck. Or use the same placement over the palm and strike (Figure 15-5B). Observe and inquire about pain. Conduct on both sides.

In a supine position use the palm/fist method to percuss the liver (Figure 15-6).

Percussion of the bladder is performed from the symphysis pubis to the umbili-

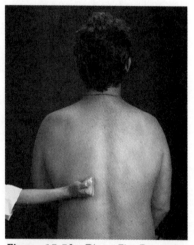

Figure 15-5A Direct Fist Percussion of the Left Kidney

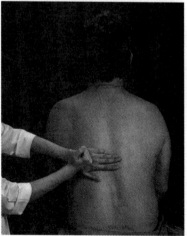

Figure 15-5B Indirect Fist Percussion of the Left Kidney

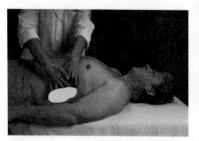

Figure 15-4 Percussion of the Spleen

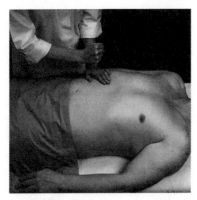

Figure 15-6   Indirect Fist Percussion of the Liver

cus. If the bladder is empty, it is not percussable above the symphysis. A full bladder sounds dull. Think about reasons for urinary retention such as medication or diabetic neuropathy, if you have asked the older adult to empty the bladder and it percusses as full.

Palpation

Pads of the fingers are used to palpate each quadrant, liver, spleen, kidney, aorta, bladder, and inguinal lymph nodes. Some nurses are not comfortable with deep palpation. Seek guidance if necessary.

Light palpation is shown in Figure 15-7. After light palpation of all four quad-

rants for masses, increased skin temperature, and tenderness, test for muscle guarding. Upon light palpation of the rectus muscle as the older adult exhales, look for guarding or tensing. If present, this may indicate peritonitis.

There are two approaches to deep palpation (see Figures 15-8 A and B).

While using the palmar surface of one hand, the other hand guides the compression (2 to 3 inches beneath the skin for deep palpation as opposed to one inch for light palpation).

Use deep palpation to all four quadrants. Note masses, location, size, consistency, pulsation, and moveability. Organs should not be enlarged unless inflammation or disease is present, such as cholecystitis or hepatitis.

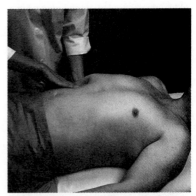

A. One-handed Method

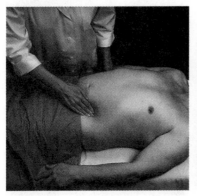

Figure 15-7   Light Palpation of the Abdomen

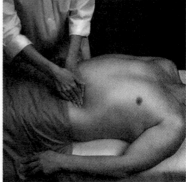

B. Bimanual Method
Figure 15-8   Deep Palpation

Palpate the liver using the bimanual method as shown in Figure 15-9.

Ask the older adult to take a deep breath; then press upward while using your other hand to support the flank. When the older adult breathes out, the liver will descend and come in contact with the hand. Practice this method on a willing colleague or significant other. Masses are abnormal.

The spleen and kidneys are palpated similarly (see Figures 15-10 and 15-11), only more gently to prevent rupture if enlarged.

Palpation of spleen and kidneys requires the older adult to breathe in, followed by palpation, ending with the client exhaling to actually feel the organ as it falls into position.

Typically the aorta is not palpated in older adults because of the remote risk of rupture.

The bladder is palpated beginning at the midline of the symphysis pubis moving upward to the umbilicus (Figure 15-12). A full bladder is smooth and round whereas an empty bladder usually is not palpable. Asymmetry may indicate a tumor.

Last, the inguinal nodes are palpated. They are located in the genital area bilat-

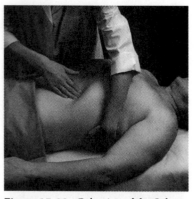

Figure 15-10   Palpation of the Spleen

⚡ NURSING ALERT

Risk for Aortic Rupture

Do not palpate an aorta that you suspect has an aneurysm. Notify the patient's physician immediately if you suspect an abdominal aortric aneurysm because the aneurysm may dissect and cause renal failure, loss of limbs, and, eventually, death if left untreated.

---

erally and are movable, small (< 1 centimeter diameter) and not painful when palpated. Large or tender nodes indicate infection, malignancy, or lymphoma.

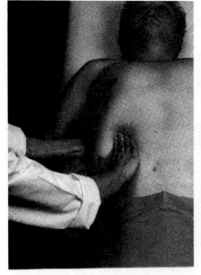

Figure 15-9   Bimanual Method

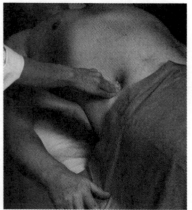

Figure 15-11   Palpation of the Right Kidney

NURSING TIPS

Incontinence (bladder or bowel) is never a normal finding in an older man or woman. Incontinence is treatable and controllable. Possible causes of urinary incontinence include infection, emotional or physiological stressors, weakened pelvic muscles, partial obstruction of the ureters, or fecal impaction. Fecal impaction, infection, obstruction, foods, or medication may cause bowel incontinence. Acceptable assessment and treatment guidelines have been established. Refer to the Appendix.

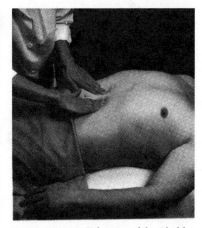

Figure 15-12 Palpation of the Bladder

References

Cauthorne-Burnette, T., & Estes, M. E. Z. (1998). *Clinical companion for health assessment and physical examination.* Albany: Delmar Publishers.

Matteson, M., McConnell, E., & Linton, A. (1997). *Gerontologic nursing: Concepts and practice.* Philadelphia: W. B. Saunders Company.

16

Assessment of Female and Male Genitalia

Key Terms

adnexa
andropause
anus
atrophic vaginitis
Bartholin's cyst
benign prostatic hypertrophy (BPH)
Candida vaginosis
cervical smear
chlamydia
Chandler's sign
clitoris
cystocele
dyspareunia
genitalia
gonorrhea
herpes simplex
hormone replacement therapy (HRT)
hydrocele
inorgasmia
Kegel exercises
leukoplakia
lithotomy
menopause
perineum
prostate-specific antigen (PSA)
rectocele
sexually transmitted diseases (STDs)
speculum
spermatocele
testicular torsion
urethral meatus
vaginal introitus

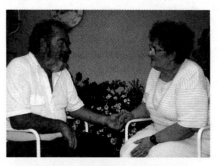

TIPS FROM THE EXPERTS

Assessment and examination of female and male **genitalia** of older adults requires skill and tact on the part of the clinician. The greater the competence and comfort of the clinician, the more at ease the older adult will feel about someone intimately examining body parts. Treating older adults as more than the sum of their body parts during a physical examination is critical to promoting human dignity. Some older adults may refuse to have their genitalia examined; it is their right to refuse. Nevertheless, it becomes the nurse's responsibility to explain, inform, describe the procedure, and allay any fear. It may be impossible to conduct this examination with the older adult who has experienced past sexual trauma or abuse or is diagnosed with dementia.

Little is known about male (or female) sexual expression in old age. Unlike females, males are able to father children well into old age (90s). Also, it is hypothesized that the incidence of homosexual behavior in older adults mirrors the rates in younger adults—5 to 10 percent. Accuracy is questionable due to the intimate nature of questions associated with sexuality. Clearly, the topic of sexuality in older adults is in dire need of investigation and research.

Assessment and evaluation of the sexual organs in older men and women require sensitive interactions and a gentle touch. For a variety of social, religious, and cultural reasons, there is a certain stigma and fear surrounding such an intimate examination. It is the nurse's responsibility to emphasize that the exam can uncover cancers and other life-threatening diseases and save one's life.

Client History and Age-Related Changes

Recent history of bleeding (vaginal, rectal, or penile) should be noted, and further diagnostic tests must be conducted. Previous pregnancies, live births, sexually transmitted diseases (**STDs**) and associated treatment regimen, infections, cancer, cysts, prostate problems, incontinence, and surgeries such as hysterectomy should be noted. Progression of menopause and associated treatment, such as hormone replacement therapy (**HRT**), helps the nurse understand and appreciate this significant transition in a woman's life. Although men do not experience menopause, testosterone levels decrease with age. **Andropause** is the term used to describe the normal hormonal decline in men. Hormonal changes in men and women begin in their 40s, although the average age for menopause is 51.

Sexual activity and sexual preference (heterosexual, homosexual, or bisexual) are important data to obtain. Sexual preferences, sexual difficulties, numbers of partners, level of interest, and presence of dyspareunia and inorgasmia are identified and discussed. Never presume that older adults have no interest in sex. Sexual expression is integral to being human.

Table 16-1 summarizes age-related changes in hormones and genitalia of older adults. Note that incontinence and impotence signal pathologies requiring treatment. Incontinence and impotence are not part of normal aging.

Anatomical landmarks of females and males are shown in Figures 16-1 through 16-3.

Assessment of the Female Genitalia

If the nurse has access to an examination table, assist the woman into a **lithotomy** position with heels in stirrups. Due to reduced flexibility and limited range of motion, this may not be feasible. Supine with knees flexed may be realistic. During a home visit, the person's bed may be used. Lighting is critical. A gooseneck lamp or flashlight is appropriate. Offer a hand-held mirror to the woman and help position it. Some clients prefer to view their exam. This encourages them to feel increased involvement and control.

Inspect pubic hair, presence of parasites, skin condition, **clitoris, urethral meatus, vaginal introitus, perineum,** and **anus.**

Don gloves and observe pubic hair. Pubic hair thins out in both males and females as hormones diminish. If flecks of blood or white particles attached to pubic hair are observed, lice or nits may be present.

Separate the labia majora with index finger and thumb. Observe color. Ecchymosis, edema, rash, nodules, or lesions are abnormal findings. Small, few cysts are within normal limits. They appear yellow, measure less than 1 centimeter, and are not painful. Some abnormal findings include **Bartholin's cyst,** infection, trauma, contact dermatitis, **herpes simplex,** varicose veins, and genital warts. Odor may indicate infection or self-care deficit related to inability to perform personal

Table 16-1   Age-Related Changes in Hormones and Specific Sexual Organs

Women:
↓ estrogen and ↓ progesterone
vaginal tissue atrophies
↓ vaginal secretions during arousal
thinning of vaginal wall
↓ vaginal lining elasticity
shrinkage of vagina and external genitalia
↑ risk for pruritis and vaginal infections

Men:
↓ testosterone
prostatic hypertrophy
↓ sperm production
↓ testicular volume
↓ intensity of ejaculation
↑ stimulation needed for erection

hygiene activities due to reduced range of motion or visual, olfactory, and tactile deterioration.

Observe the clitoris and urethral meatus by separating the labia minora. In fleshier individuals and due to sagging of the skin, it may be initially difficult to locate and distinguish the clitoris from the urethral meatus. The clitoris is 0.50 to 1 centimeter in diameter, and should be free of discharge or lesions.

The urethral meatus is below the clitoris. Discharge, redness, or swelling indicates a possible urinary tract infection (UTI), Skene's gland infection, carcinoma, or urethral caruncle.

While the labia minora is retracted, inspect the opening to the vagina (vaginal introitus), which should appear shiny, unobstructed, and odorless. Dryness and atrophy are not uncommon in older women. Anything other than white or clear discharge is abnormal, indicating infections

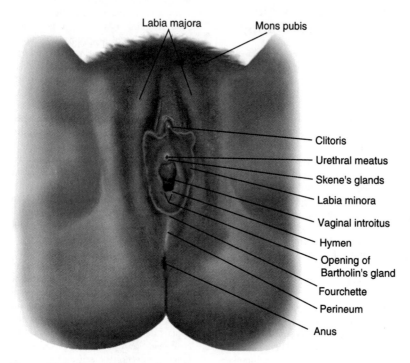

Figure 16-1   External Female Genitalia

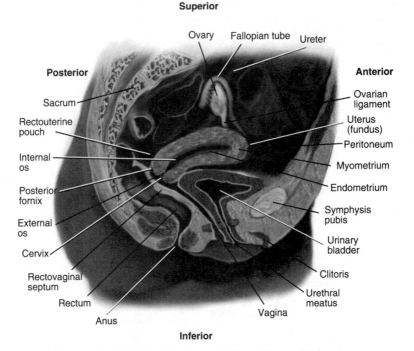

Figure 16-2   Left-sided Sagittal Section at Midline of Internal Pelvic Organs

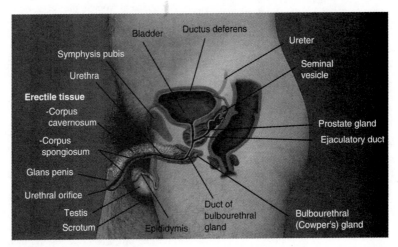

Figure 16-3   Male Genitalia

such as gonorrhea, Chalamydia, *Candida* vaginosis, or **atrophic vaginitis.** Bulging of the anterior vaginal wall suggests a **cystocele.** A history of multiple births, obesity, and lack of HRT predispose women to cystocele, **rectocele** (bulging of posterior vaginal wall and part of rectum), and incontinence, yet none of these conditions is part of the normal aging process.

Observe the perineum and anus. Both should appear smooth and darker than the surrounding skin. Some skin tags in the area are within normal limits. External hemorrhoids are a common findings. When they are excessively large, they interfere with comfort and bowel elimination. Treatment is warranted.

Palpation of the External Genitalia

Palpate the labia. Swelling, pain, and asymmetry indicate infection. "Milk" the urethra by inserting the index finger into the vagina anteriorly as shown in Figure 16-4. There should be no pain or discharge.

Test for vaginal muscle tone by asking the woman to squeeze muscles while your finger is in the vagina. Reduced muscle tone can be improved through **Kegel exercises,** a controlled tightening and releasing of vaginal, perineal, and rectal muscles. Test for perineal strength by turning your finger posterior to the perineum, then asking the woman to squeeze muscles in the vaginal area. The perineum should feel smooth throughout.

Speculum Examination of Internal Genitalia

Explain the procedure to the woman. Some older women may be nervous or may not know what to expect. Women who have not had access to adequate health care may never have had experienced such an exam. Remember that cultural and religious beliefs play an important role in whether the woman is agreeable to such an intimate procedure.

A Graves' bivalve speculum is useful for examining most women. Warm and lubricate the speculum. Hold the speculum with your dominant hand with blades closed. Open the vagina by using index and middle fingers, and place the speculum at an oblique angle into the vagina. See Figure 16-5A and 16-5B

After the speculum is inserted, withdraw the fingers of the nondominant hand. Rotate the speculum into a horizontal position and then at a 45-degree angle against the posterior vaginal wall until the end of the speculum is positioned at the end of the vagina. Depress the lever, opening the blades. Inspect the cervix for color, shape, position, size, lesions, and discharge. In postmenopausal women, the cervix is not as shiny, appearing pale pink. Bright red indicates inflammation or infection. Normal size of the cervix is approximately 2 to 5 centimeters. Shapes of the cervical os are shown in Figure 16-6.

Collecting Specimens

In this order, cytological smears and cultures are collected: **Papanicolaou (PAP)** smear, chlamydial, gonococcal, and any other specimens. The smears are obtained while the speculum is in place.

For the PAP test, insert the cytobrush through the speculum 1 centimeter into the cervical os. With thumb and index finger, roll the brush 360 degrees and then counterclockwise. Remove the brush and

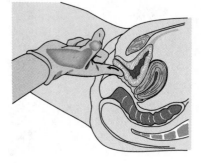

Figure 16-4   Milking the Urethra

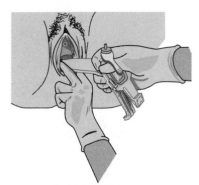

A. Opening of the Vaginal Introitus

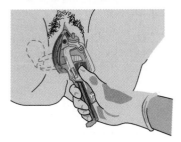

B. Opening of the Speculum Blades
Figure 16-5   Speculum Examination

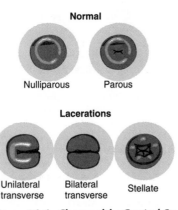

Figure 16-6   Shapes of the Cervical Os

gently spread the cells on the part of the slide marked *E* (if using a sectional slide).

Obtain a **cervical smear** by using the split end of the Ayre spatula. Insert into the speculum. Insert the longer portion into the cervical os. Rotate once and smear on the slide labeled *C,* if a sectional slide is used.

A vaginal pool smear is obtained by inserting the opposite end (rounded) of the Ayre spatula into the posterior vaginal fornix and gently scraping the area. Remove and spread gently onto the slide section marked *V.* Spray the entire slide with cytological fixative and follow guidelines for sending it to the lab. Reportable findings comprise benign cellular changes, atypical squamous cell of undetermined significance, and epithelial cell abnormalities indicative of infection or more serious cellular and tissue changes.

To test for *Neisseria gonorrhoeae,* insert a sterile swab applicator into the cervical

os. Hold for 30 seconds. Remove and smear in a *Z* pattern on a Thayer-Martin culture plate. Send to the lab per their guidelines.

Prepare a saline mount or "wet prep"

🕊 NURSING ALERT

Risk Factors for Female Genitalia Cancer

Cervical Cancer
- Early age at first intercourse
- Multiple sex partners
- Prior history of human papillomavirus
- Tobacco use
- Family history

Endometrial Cancer
- Early or late menarche (before age 11 or after age 16)
- History of infertility
- Failure to ovulate
- Unopposed estrogen therapy
- Use of tamoxifen
- Obesity
- Family history

Ovarian Cancer
- Advancing age
- Nulliparity
- History of breast cancer
- Family history of ovarian cancer

Vaginal Cancer
- Daughters of women who ingested DES during pregnancy

slide to observe for white blood cells (WBCs). Take a cervicovaginal specimen and spread on a microscopic slide. Add one drop of normal saline and a cover slip. Greater than 10 WBCs per field suggests infection.

For the KOH prep tests for overgrowth of yeast *(Candida)*, a cervicovaginal specimen is obtained and spread on a microscopic slide. One drop of potassium hydroxide is added, followed by a cover slip. When visualized under a microscope, chains of budding yeast suggest a *Candida* infection.

The final step after taking the above specimens is swabbing the cervix with 5% acetic acid wash. No change is normal, whereas blanching implies presence of human papillomavirus (the virus that causes genital warts). Table 16-2 lists specimens for cytological smears.

An anal culture is obtained by inserting a sterile cotton swab applicator 1 centimeter into the rectum. Remove any feces, if present, and start over. Hold applicator in the rectum for 30 seconds. Remove and smear in *Z* motion on a Thayer-Martin culture plate. Absence of *Neisseria gonorrhoeae* is normal.

While removing the opened, unlocked speculum, observe the vaginal wall, which should appear pale pink without lesions and redness. **Leukoplakia,** which appears as white specks on the vaginal wall, may suggest *Candida.*

Table 16-2 Cytological Smears/Specimens

PAP smear
Cervical smear
Vaginal pool smear
Gonococcal culture specimen
Saline mount or "wet prep"
KOH prep (for *Candida*)
5% acetic acid wash (for human papillomavirus)

Summarized from Cauthorne-Burnette, T., & Estes, M. E. Z. (1998). *Clinical companion for health assessment and physical examination.* Albany: Delmar Publishers.

Bimanual Examination

Explain each step of the "internal exam." Some older women postpone a GYN exam because of avoidance of such manipulation of the genitals. Inform them that some bleeding after the exam is normal. Always reassure the woman that the health benefit reaped from the exam far outweighs the temporary discomfort and embarrassment.

Use water-soluble lubricant on the fingers of your dominant hand. Stand between the woman's legs while she remains in the lithotomy position. Insert index and middle fingers halfway into the vagina, with finger pads up. Press down gently on the posterior wall of the vagina. Reaffirm to the woman that she should feel some pressure. Insert the entire length of the index and middle fingers and slowly palpate the vaginal wall, which should feel smooth. Lesions, although abnormal, are most commonly found on the upper one-third of the posterior vaginal wall.

Next, palpate the cervix with the palmar surface of the hands facing upward. The nondominant hand is placed on the abdomen between the umbilicus and symphysis pubis. Consistency, position, shape, tenderness, and mobility are determined. With your two inserted fingers, grasp the cervix and move it gently side to side to assess for mobility. The woman should experience a negative **Chandler's sign** (no pain upon palpation). See Figure 16-7, which illustrates cervical mobility.

Palpate around the fornices, which should feel smooth. Abnormal findings include malignancies or polyps. Palpate the uterus by gently pushing the pelvic organs out of the way, and stabilize using the nondominant hand already on the abdomen. Press that hand down and try to palpate the uterus between your hands. See Figure 16-8.

The uterus should feel nontender, smooth, and firm, without masses. It is not uncommon to fail to palpate the uterus in an older woman because of shrinkage and atrophy.

Fallopian tubes and ovaries are rarely palpable in an older woman. Palpation be-

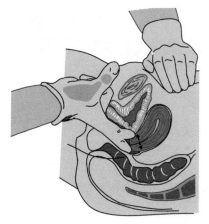

Figure 16-7 Assessment of Cervical Mobility

tween the dominant (inserted) and nondominant fingers at the right and left quadrants inside the anterior iliac spine may capture the ovary. Normally the **adnexa** (ovaries and Fallopian tube structures) are almond-shaped, mobile, and smooth, without tenderness. Pain is a warning sign of a cyst or tumor. Refer to Figure 16-9 for this procedure.

Rectovaginal Exam

Withdraw fingers from the vagina and change gloves. Explain the procedure. Lubricate the index and middle fingers of the dominant hand. Ask the woman to bear down, which relaxes the anal sphincter. Insert the index and middle fingers into the vagina and rectum, respectively. Anal sphincter tone may be affected by medications such as benzodiazepines, which relax sphincter muscles. See Figure 16-10.

Palpate, with help from the nondominant hand on the abdomen, and assess the following:

• Rectovaginal septum for patency
• Cervix and uterus for posterior lesions
• Rectouterine pouch for lesions

If stool is present, test for occult blood. Prepare a warm washcloth for the woman to clean herself, or assist if necessary. Palpate for hernias.

After the entire examination, apprise the woman that some bleeding is normal. Dignity is important. A smiling, supportive face, and nurturing body language compensate for any depersonalization that the

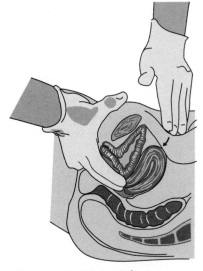

Figure 16-8 Uterine Palpation

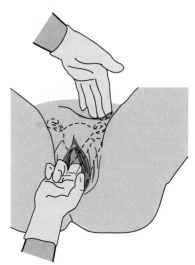

Figure 16-9 Palpation of the Left Adnexa

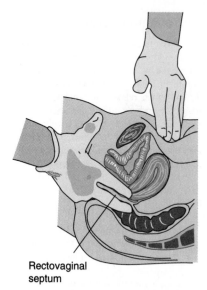

Rectovaginal
septum

Figure 16-10　Rectovaginal Exam

Table 16-3　Sexual History Specific to the Older Adult Male

Medical history of:
- STDs
- UTIs
- Prostatitis
- Trauma
- Epididymitis
- Cancer
- Benign prostatic hypertrophy (BPH)
- Premature ejaculation
- Impotence
- Infertility
- Mother's use of hormones during pregnancy (diethylstilbestrol [DES])

Surgical history of:
- Prostatectomy
- Transurethral prostatectomy
- Circumcision
- Vasectomy
- Hernia repair
- Testicular surgery for malpositioning of testicles
- Lesion removal

Social history of:
- Drug usage (cocaine, barbiturates, amphetamines)
- Number of partners
- Frequency and types of sexual expression
- Condom use
- Sexual preferences
- Perception of sexual satisfaction

woman may have felt or perceived during the exam. Reinforce that her actions *today* are lifesaving measures. In addition, don't rush after the exam. Stiffness from being in the lithotomy position is normal.

Assessment of Male Genitalia

Although many experts feel the mind is the most powerful sexual organ, healthy genitalia, overall physical mobility, and flexibility are also needed for sexual expression. Figure 16-3 displays the anatomy of the male genitalia.

Assessment of male genitalia and sexuality incorporates pertinent medical/surgical history, family health, and social history. See Table 16-3.

Inspection of the Male Genitalia

While the male client is in a supine position, inspect hair distribution, penis, scrotum, urethral meatus, and inguinal area. Pubic hair will appear thinned out in an older male. No swelling, inflammation, or lesions should be present. Ask the man to retract the foreskin of the penis. Look for any inflammation, swelling, or discharge. It is not uncommon (and normal) to note the dorsal vein. Penises vary in shape and size, as well as in diameter and length. Unless there are signs and symptoms of infection or gross asymmetry is present, variations in shape are normal. Presence of chancres may indicate syphilis *(Treponema palidum)*, genital warts, or other STDs. Classic signs of infection include:

- discharge from the penis
- scrotal or testicular pain
- difficulties with urination
- lesions on the penis

Some abnormalities are summarized in Table 16-4.

Move the penis to the side and inspect the scrotum for swelling, lesions, and redness. The scrotal skin is slightly darker than surrounding skin, and is smooth and flaccid in the older male. Locate the urethral meatus. There should be no redness or discharge. Culture any discharge. Palpate the penis between thumb and index finger. The male client should feel no pain. Refer to Figure 16-11.

Palpate the right, then left, testicle using the thumb and first two fingers. Palpation should not cause pain. Testicles should be symmetric. Locate the epididymis, which is comma-shaped. Locate the spermatic cord, which should feel smooth and round. Abnormalities include **hydrocele** (a large, pear-sized mass filled with fluid) and **spermatocele** (cystic mass in epididymis or testis). **Testicular torsion** is a twisting of the testis causing venous and possibly arterial obstruction and edema. Upon palpation, pain and sensitivity will be experienced. Refer to Figures 16-12 and 16-13.

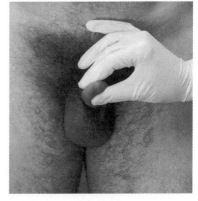

Figure 16-11 Palpation of the Urethral Meatus

Findings of a smaller, soft testicle is associated with estrogen therapy in the older male. Also, scrotal edema may be present

⚕ NURSING ALERT

Warning Signs of STDs in the Male Patient

- Bloody or purulent penile discharge
- Scrotal and/or testicular pain
- Burning and/or pain on urination
- Penile lesion

Table 16-4   Some Abnormalities of the Penis

Chancre	Primary syphilis
Chancroid, papular lesion	*Haemophilus ducreyi*
Condyloma acuminatum	Genital warts (pinhead lesions or larger groupings)
Maculopapular lesions; tan, brown, pink, white, violet	Neoplasm
Vesicular lesions, pustular	Herpes simplex
Candida	Flat, white pustules, moist sites
Tinea cruris	Reddened plaques with scaling: fungal infection
Paraphimosis	Retracted foreskin unable to return to its original position
Priapism	Continued uncontrollable erection: leukemia, cancers
Penile curvature (chordee)	Congenital cause: cause unknown

with congestive heart failure (CHF) and portal vein obstruction.

Observe for inguinal swelling or bulges suggestive of hernia. Ask the male client to stand and bear down. The inguinal area may have less muscle tone, yet both sides should be symmetric. Next, ask the male client to bear down while you palpate the skin over the inguinal and femoral areas for lymph nodes. Use the index and middle fingers and follow the right scrotal sac to the spermatic cord until you reach a slit-like opening (external inguinal ring). With the finger pad facing upward, advance toward the inguinal canal and ask the male client to cough. Feel for masses. Repeat on the left side. No masses or bulges should be present, although lymph nodes of 1 centimeter are a normal finding. Enlarged lymph nodes suggest infection. See Figure 16-14.

Table 16-5 lists warning signs of hernia, which every man should know.

Figures 16-15, 16-16, and 16-17 illustrate indirect, direct, and femoral canal hernias.

Auscultate the scrotum if a mass is found. This is done by placing the stethoscope over the scrotal mass while the male client is in a supine position. No bowel sounds should be heard. With an indirect inguinal hernia it is possible to hear bowel sounds because of the herniation of bowel extending into the scrotum. The client will need immediate surgery.

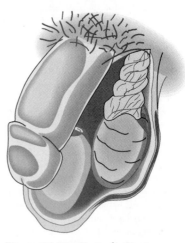

Figure 16-13   Testicular Torsion

Examination of the Anus, Rectum, and Prostate

The anorectum and prostate exam is essential to maintaining and screening for health problems in men to prevent rectal

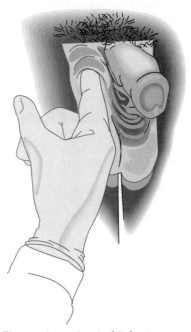

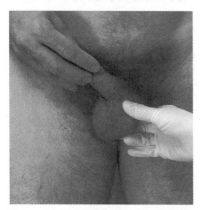

Figure 16-12   Palpation of the Testicle

Figure 16-14   Inguinal Palpation

Table 16-5   Warning Signs of Hernia

- Bulging in the groin area, especially upon exertion
- Scrotal or inguinal mass
- Discomfort in the inguinal or scrotal area
- Self-treatment of support girdle

*If any of the above is present, refer the male client for further testing.

and prostate cancer, which increases as men pass their 50s. Important anatomical landmarks are shown in Figures 16-18 and 16-19.

The prostate gland is located against the anterior rectal wall. It is approximately the size of a chestnut (3 cm x 3 cm) and has ducts that feed into the urethra. There are five lobes to the prostate, two of which can be palpated, the right and left lateral lobes. The other three lobes are the anterior, posterior, and median lobes.

Inspection

After explaining the entire procedure, inspect the perineum, sacrococcygeal areas, and anal mucosa while the male client is

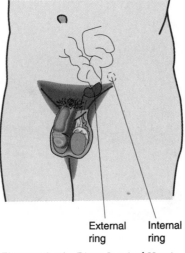

External ring   Internal ring

Figure 16-16   Direct Inguinal Hernia

in one of three positions indicated in Figures 16-20A, B, and C.

Swelling, lesions, redness, and inflammation are abnormal findings. Psoriasis, *Candida,* pruritis, or pilonidal cyst over the sacral region are not within normal limits and warrant investigation.

Spread buttocks apart to inspect the anus. The anus is normally darker than the sur-

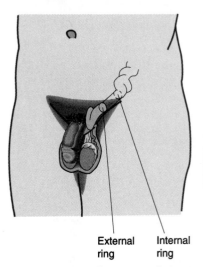

External ring   Internal ring

Figure 16-15   Indirect Inguinal Hernia

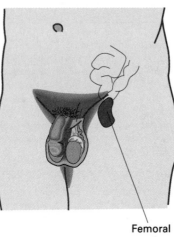

Femoral canal

Figure 16-17   Femoral Hernia

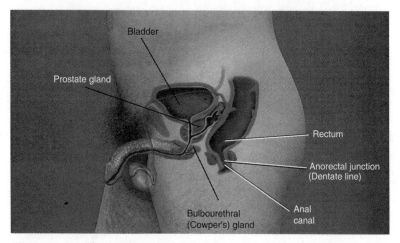

Figure 16-18   The Anorectum and Prostate

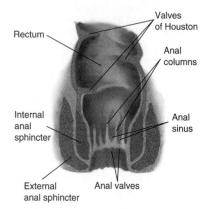

Figure 16-19   Anal Canal

rounding skin, and should be free of lesions, swelling, inflammation, or bleeding. Bluish, grape-like lumps at the anus indicate hemorrhoids. An anal fissure or tear may indicate some type of trauma (anal manipulation or intercourse). See Figure 16-21. Exudate from the anus indicates abscess, infection such as herpes simplex, or gonococcal proctitis.

Palpation of Anus and Rectum

Explain that sensations of urination and defecation are normal. Lubricate the gloved index finger of your dominant hand and place the fingertip at the anal orifice. As the male client bears down, insert finger gently at a 45-degree angle,

never at 90 degrees. The sphincter should relax. Then insert the entire finger. Assess for sphincter tone. See Figure 16-22 and 16-23.

Palpate all sides of the rectum by moving the breadth of the finger along the rectal wall. Do not move your finger in and out, but move around lateral, anterior, and posterior walls. Any bulges, masses, tenderness, or nodules should be noted in terms of size and exact location. Possible causes of internal masses and nodules include rectal polyps, internal hemorrhoids,

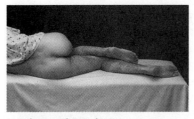

A. Left Lateral Decubitus

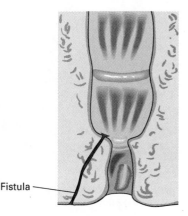

Fistula

Figure 16-21 Anorectal Fistula

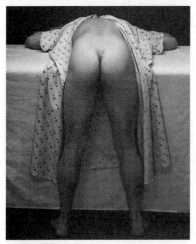

B. Standing

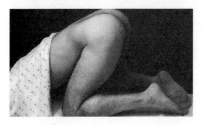

C. Knee-Chest
Figure 16-20 Patient Positions for the Anus, Rectum, and Prostate Examination

an enlarged prostate due to increased levels of dihydrotestosterone, which generates cell growth. Tables 16-6 and 16-7 summarize risk factors and prevention for prostate cancer and risk factors, and prevention for rectal cancer. Both can be prevented if nurses and doctors make a point of early screening.

Withdraw your finger and test any stool for occult blood. Offer the man a warm washcloth and assist with cleaning if necessary.

fecal impaction, anal cancer or rectal prolapse. See Figure 16-24.

Palpate the prostate by inserting the lubricated finger of your dominant hand into the rectum as shown in Figure 16-25.

The prostate gland should feel smooth, small, mobile, and nontender. Firm, hard nodules on the prostate may indicate cancer. Benign prostatic hypertrophy (BPH) is

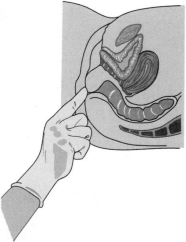

Figure 16-22 Position of the Index Finger for Anorectal Palpation

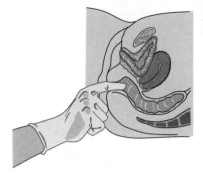

Figure 16-23 Position of the Index Finger in the Anorectum

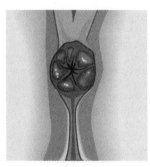

Figure 16-24 Rectal Prolapse

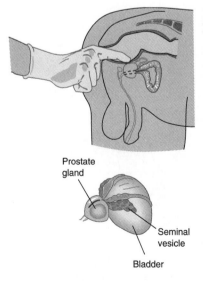

Prostate gland

Seminal vesicle

Bladder

Figure 16-25 Prostatic Palpation

Table 16-6   Risk Factors and Prevention of Prostate Cancer

Risk factors:
- Men > 50 years of age
- Having a direct relative (sibling or father) with prostate cancer
- African American
- High levels of serum testosterone

Prostate cancer prevention:
- Annual digital rectal exam
- **PSA (prostate-specific antigen)** recommended by some professional groups annually
- Referral to a urologist for further screening based on abnormal findings in the above

Summarized from Abrams, W. B., Beers, M. H., Berkow, R. & Fletcher, A. J. (Eds). *The Merck manual of geriatrics* (2nd ed.). (1995). Whitehouse Station: Merck Research Laboratories.

Table 16-7   Risk Factors and Prevention for Rectal Cancer

Risk factors:
- Over 55 years old
- Family history of colorectal cancer
- For women: history of ovarian, endometrial, or breast cancer
- Inflammatory bowel disease
- Diet low in fiber, high in animal fat

Prevention:
- Routine sigmoidoscopy after 50 years old
- Colonoscopy at 50 and every 5 years therafter
- Annual fecal occult blood testing
- Annual digital rectal exam

Summarized from *The Merck manual of geriatrics,* 1995. Whitehouse Station: Merck Research Laboratories

References

Abrams, W. B., Beers, M. H., Berkow, R., & Fletcher A. J. (Eds.). *The Merck manual of geriatrics* (2nd ed.) (1995). Whitehouse Station: Merck Research Laboratories.

Cauthorne-Burnette, T., & Estes, M. E. Z. (1998). *Clinical companion for health assessment and physical examination.* Albany: Delmar Publishers.

Appendix A

GENERAL
Client's perception of general state of health at the present, difference from usual state, vitality and energy levels

NEUROLOGICAL
Headache, change in balance, incoordination, loss of movement, change in sensory perception/feeling in an extremity, change in speech, change in smell, fainting (syncope), loss of memory, tremors, involuntary movement, loss of consciousness, seizures, weakness, head injury

PSYCHOLOGICAL
Irritability, nervousness, tension, increased stress, difficulty concentratiing, mood changes, suicidal thoughts, depression.

SKIN
Rashes, itching, changes in skin pigmentation, black and blue marks (ecchymoses), change in color or size of mole, sores, lumps, change in skin texture, odors, excessive sweating, acne, loss of hair (alopecia), excessive growth of hair or growth of hair in unusual locations (hirsutism), change in nails, amount of time spent in the sun

EYES
Blurred vision, visual acuity, glasses, contacts, sensitivity to light (photophobia), excessive tearing, night blindness, double vision (diplopia), drainage, bloodshot eyes, pain, blind spots, flashing lights, halos around objects, glaucoma, cataracts

EARS
Hearing deficits, hearing aid, pain, discharge, lightheadedness (vertigo), ringing in the ears (tinnitus), earaches, infection

NOSE AND SINUSES
Frequent colds, discharge, itching, hay fever, postnasal drip, stuffiness, sinus pain, polyps, obstruction, nosebleed (epistaxis), change in sense of smell

MOUTH
Toothache, tooth abscess, dentures, bleeding/swollen gums, difficulty chewing, sore tongue, change in taste, lesions, change in salivation, bad breath

THROAT/NECK
Hoarseness, change in voice, frequent sore throats, difficulty swallowing, pain/stiffness, enlarged thyroid (goiter)

continued

RESPIRATORY
Shortness of breath (dyspnea), shortness of breath on exertion, phlegm (sputum), cough, sneezing, wheezing, coughing up blood (hemoptysis), frequent upper respiratory tract infections, pneumonia, emphysema, asthma, tuberculosis

CARDIOVASCULAR
Shortness of breath that wakes you up in the night (paroxysmal nocturnal dyspnea), chest pain, heart murmur, palpitations, fainting (syncope), sleep on pillows to breathe better (orthopnea; state number of pillows used), swelling (edema), cold hands/feet, leg cramps, myocardial infarction, hypertension, valvular disease, pain in calf when walking (intermittent claudication), varicose veins, inflammation of a vein (thrombophlebitis), blood clot in leg (deep vein thrombosis), anemia

BREASTS
Pain, tenderness, discharge, lumps, change in size, dimpling

GASTROINTESTINAL
Change in appetite, nausea, vomiting, diarrhea, constipation, usual bowel habits, black tarry stools (melena), vomiting blood (hematemesis), change in stool color, excessive gas (flatulence), belching, regurgitation, heartburn, difficulty swallowing (dysphagia), abdominal pain, jaundice, hemorrhoids, hepatitis, peptic ulcers, gallstones

URINARY
Change in urine color, voiding habits, painful urination (dysuria), hesitancy, urgency, frequency, excessive urination at night (nocturia), increased urine volume (polyuria), dribbling, loss in force of stream, bedwetting, change in urine volume, incontinence, pain in lower abdomen (suprapubic pain), kidney stones, urinary tract infections

MUSCULOSKELETAL
Joint stiffness, muscle pain, back pain, limitation of movement, redness, swelling, weakness, bony deformity, broken bones, dislocations, sprains, gout, arthritis, osteoporosis, herniated disc

FEMALE REPRODUCTIVE
Vaginal discharge, change in libido, infertility, sterility, pain during intercourse, menses: last menstrual period (LMP), age period started (menarche), regularity, duration, amount of bleeding, premenstrual symptoms, intermenstrual bleeding, painful periods (dysmenorrhea), menopause: age of onset, duration, symptoms, bleeding, obstetrical: number of pregnancies, number of miscarriages/abortions, number of children, type of delivery, complications, type of birth control, estrogen therapy

MALE REPRODUCTIVE
Change in libido, infertility, sterility, impotence, pain during intercourse, age at onset of puberty, testicular pain, penile discharge, erections, emissions, hernias, enlarged prostate, type of birth control

NUTRITION
Present weight, usual weight, food intolerances, food likes/dislikes, where meals are eaten

continued

ENDOCRINE

Bulging eyes, fatigue, change in size of head, hands, or feet, weight change, heat/cold intolerances, excessive sweating, increased thirst, increased hunger, change in body hair distribution, swelling in the anterior neck, diabetes mellitus

LYMPH NODES

Enlargement, tenderness

HEMATOLOGICAL

Easy bruising/bleeding, anemia, sickle cell anemia, blood type

From *Health Assessment and Physical Examination* by M.E. Z. 1998, Estes, Albany, NY: Delmar Publishers. Adapted with permission.

Appendix B

Test	Age-Related Change	Geriatric Value
Hemoglobin	Slightly decreased, related to reduced hematopoiesis	M: 10–17 g/100 ml F: 9–17 g/100 ml
Hematocrit	Slightly decreased, related to reduced hematopoiesis	M: 38%–54% F: 35%–49%
Leukocytes	Decreased, related to decreased T & B lymphocytes	3,100–9,000 cu mm
Sedimentation rate	Slightly increased	Less than 22 mm/hr
Albumin	Decreased, related to reduced liver size and enzyme production	M: 2.3–4.7 g/100 ml F: 2.6–5.0 g/100/ml
Alkaline phosphatase	Increased, related to decreased liver function	M: 21.3–80.8 units F: 19.9–83.4 units
Blood urea nitrogen	Increased, related to compromised renal function	M: 8–35 mg/100 ml F: 6–30 mg/100 ml
Creatinine	Increased	0.4–1.9 mg/100 ml
Calcium	Slightly decreased	9–10.9 mg/100 ml
Glucose	Increased	140 mg/100 ml
Potassium	Increased	3.0–5.9 MEQ/L
Creatinine clearance	Must be calculated to consider decreased glomerular filtration rate	
Men		(140 – age) x kg body weight divided by 72
Women		(140 – age) x kg body weight x 0.85 divided by 72

(Adapted from Ham & Sloane, 1992; Hogstel & Keen-Payne, 1996).

Appendix C

Braden Pressure Ulcer Risk Assessment[1]

Patient Name _____

Age _____ Address _____

Date _____

(Indicate appropriate numbers below)
NOTE: Bed- and chairbound individuals with impaired ability to reposition themselves should
be assessed for risk of developing pressure ulcers.
Patients with established pressure ulcers should be reassessed periodically.

SENSORY PERCEPTION ability to respond meaningfully to pressure-related discomfort	1. Completely Limited: Unresponsive (does not moan, flinch, or grasp) to painful stimuli, due to diminished level of consciousness or sedation. OR limited ability to feel pain over most of body surface.	2. Very Limited: Responds only to painful stimuli. Cannot communicate discomfort except by moaning or restlessness. OR has a sensory impairment which limits the ability to feel pain or discomfort over 1/2 of body.	3. Slightly Limited: Responds to verbal commands, but cannot always communicate discomfort or need to be turned. OR has some sensory impairment which limits ability to feel pain or discomfort in 1 or 2 extremities.	4. No Impairment: Responds to verbal commands, has no sensory deficit which would limit ability to feel or voice pain or discomfort.	
MOISTURE degree to which skin is exposed to moisture	1. Constantly Moist: Skin is kept moist almost constantly by perspiration, urine, etc. Dampness is detected every time patient is moved or turned.	2. Very Moist: Skin is often, but not always, moist. Linen must be changed at least once a shift.	3. Occasionally Moist: Skin is occasionally moist, requiring an extra linen change approximately once a day.	4. Rarely Moist: Skin is usually dry, linen only requires changing at routine intervals.	
ACTIVITY degree of physical activity	1. Bedfast: Confined to bed.	2. Chairfast: Ability to walk severely limited or non-existent. Cannot bear own weight and/or must be assisted into chair or wheelchair.	3. Walks Occasionally: Walks occasionally during day, but for very short distances, with or without assistance. Spends majority of each shift in bed or chair.	4. Walks Frequently: Walks outside the room at least twice a day and inside room at least once every 2 hours during waking hours.	
MOBILITY ability to change and control body position	1. Completely Immobile: Does not make even slight changes in body or extremity position without assistance.	2. Very Limited: Makes occasional slight changes in body or extremity position but unable to make frequent or significant changes independently.	3. Slightly Limited: Makes frequent though slight changes in body or extremity position independently.	4. No Limitations: Makes major and frequent changes in position without assistance.	
NUTRITION usual food intake pattern	1. Very Poor: Never eats a complete meal. Rarely eats more than 1/3 of any food offered. Eats 2 servings or less of protein (meat or dairy products) per day. Takes fluids poorly. Does not take a liquid dietary supplement. OR is NPO and/or maintained on clear liquids or IV's for more than 5 days.	2. Probably Inadequate: Rarely eats a complete meal and generally eats only about 1/2 of any food offered. Protein intake includes only 3 servings of meat or dairy products per day. Occasionally will take a dietary supplement. OR receives less than optimum amount of liquid diet or tube feeding.	3. Adequate: Eats over half of most meals. Eats a total of 4 servings of protein (meat, dairy products) each day. Occasionally will refuse a meal, but will usually take a supplement if offered. OR is on a tube feeding or TPN regimen which probably meets most of nutritional needs.	4. Excellent: Eats most of every meal. Never refuses a meal. Usually eats a total of 4 or more servings of meat and dairy products. Occasionally eats between meals. Does not require supplementation.	
FRICTION AND SHEAR	1. Problem: Requires moderate to maximum assistance in moving. Complete lifting without sliding against sheets is impossible. Frequently slides down in bed or chair, requiring frequent repositioning with maximum assistance. Spasticity, contractures or agitation lead to almost constant friction.	2. Potential Problem: Moves feebly or requires minimum assistance. During a move skin probably slides to some extent against sheets, chair, restraints, or other devices. Maintains relatively good position in chair or bed most of the time but occasionally slides down.	3. No Apparent Problem: Moves in bed and in chair independently and has sufficient muscle strength to lift up completely during move. Maintains good position in bed or chair at all times.		
NOTE: Patients with a total score of 16 or less are considered to be at risk of developing pressure ulcers. (15 or 16 = low risk, 13 or 14 = moderate risk, 12 or less = high risk)				TOTAL SCORE:	

1. Braden BI, Bergstrom N. Clinical utility of the Braden Scale for Predicting Pressure Sore Risk. *Decubitus.* 1989;2:44-51.

Appendix D

U.S. Department of Health and Human Services. (1994). *Nutritional assessment of patient with pressure ulcer(s)* AHCPR Publication No. 95-0653). Rockville, MD: Author.

Appendix E

Pressure Ulcer Care by Risk Factors

Risk Factor	Preventive Actions

1. Bed or Chair Confinement	• Inspect skin at least once a day
	• Bathe when needed for comfort or cleanliness.
	• Prevent dry skin.
	• For a person in bed:
	  1. Change position at least every 2 hours.
	  2. Use a special mattress that contains foam, air, gel, or water
	  3. Raise the head of bed as little and for as short a time as possible.
	• For a person in a chair:
	  1. Change position every hour.
	  2. Use foam, gel, or air cushion to relieve pressure
	• Reduce friciton by:
	  1. Lifting rather than dragging when repositioning
	  2. Using corn starch on skin.
	• Avoid use of donut-shape cushions.
	• Participate in a rehabilitation program.

2. Inability to Move	• Persons confined to chairs should be repositioned every hour if unable to do so themselves. • For a person in a chair who is able to shift his or her own weight, change position at least every 15 minutes. • Use pillows or wedges to keep knees or ankles from touching each other. • When in bed, place pillow under legs from mid-calf to ankle to keep heels off the bed.

3. Loss of Bowel or Bladder Control	• Clean skin as soon as soiled.
	• Assess and treat urine leaks.
	• If moisture cannot be controlled:
	  1. Use absorbent pads and/or briefs with a quick-drying surface.
	  2. Protect skin with a cream or ointment.

4. Poor Nutrition	• Eat a balanced diet. • If a normal diet is not possible, talk to health care provider about nutritional supplements.
5. Lowered Mental Awareness	• Choose preventive actions that apply to the the person with lowered mental awareness. For example, if the person is chair-bound, refer to the specific preventive actions outlined in Risk Factor 1.

Appendix F

Assessment step	Process/details
1. Question client about incontinence	"Do you have trouble holding your urine?" "Do you ever wear a pad?" "Do you ever experience dribbling or loss of urine when you don't want to?"
2. Investigate clients who complain of incontinence	Follow through on client complaints.
3. Evaluate client:	
A. History	• Find out history; dimensions of medical, neurologic, genitourinary, medication review.
	• Duration and characteristics of incontinence
	• Frequency, timing, amount of continent and incontinent events
	• Elements which prompt incontinence: abdominal pressure, surgery, trauma, disease
	• Nocturia, dysuria, hesitancy, straining, interrupted stream, hematuria, pain, frequency, urgency, increased leakage
	• Fluid intake pattern
	• Change in bowel or sexual function
	• Use of pads, briefs, other devices
	• Previous treatments
B. Physical	• Abdominal exam (fullness, tenderness, masses); estimate post void residual volume (PVR) [<50 cc "normal"; >200 cc inadequate]
	• Genital exam in men (penile abnormalities)
	• Pelvic exam in women (atrophy, prolapse, weak muscle tone)
	• Rectal exam (tone, fecal impaction, masses, prostatic contour)
	• Comorbid conditions: edema, assess cognition, manual dexterity

continued

Assessment step	Process/details

C. Urinalysis
   4. Other important
       assessment data
	• Presence of bacteria, protein, blood
	• Voiding diary
	• PVR: 200cc (abnormal); 50–199cc (clinical judgement "uncertain"; <50cc (normal)
	• Provocative stress test (try to prompt incontinence)
	• Blood tests
	• Urine cytology
	• Environmental and social assessments

5. Types of incontinence	**Functional:** environmental barrier causing incontinence e.g. no call light **Stress:** urinary leakage when coughing, sneezing due to weakened pelvic muscles **Urge:** detrusor instability; spontaneous contractions of bladder; common with CNS damage, dementia, stroke **Overflow:** detrusor hyporeflexivity; loss of fullness sensation as with diabetic neuropathy **Mixed:** combination of the above and thus difficult to treat

Summarized from Urinary Incontinence Guideline Panel. *Urinary Incontinence in Adults: Quick Reference Guide for Clinicians.* AHCPR Pub. No. 92-0041. Rockville, MD: Agency for Health Care Policy and Research, Public Health Service, US Dept. of Health and Human Services, March 1992.

Appendix G

Bowel Incontinence: Factors and Assessment

Associated factors to evaluate:
- Urinary incontinence of history thereof
- Fecal impaction
- Infection
- Loss of muscle tone of the sphincter
- Medications (polypharmacy)
- Low fiber, high sugar diet
- Neurological diseases
- Immobility of poor mobility
- Severe cognitive decline
- Reduced social activities
- Age over 70 years old

Conduct abdominal, genitourinary, rectal and dietary examination.
Conduct a nutritional assessment and psychosocial assessment.
Basic labwork, stool for occult blood.
Treatment requires addressing the etiology of the incontinence.
Refer to gastroenterologist if necessary.

Adapted from Fitapatrick, J. J., Fulmer, T., Wallace, M., & Flaherty, E. *Geriatric Nursing Research Digest* (2000). "Bowel Function," E. Hermann & Zembrzuski, C.D. New York: Springer Publishing Company.

Appendix H

1. Ask about pain; client's self-report is the best source of assessment.
2. Use easy rating scales.
3. Measure pain ratings before and after initiating treatment/interventions.
4. Teach clients and families to use assessment scales.
5. When client cannot verbalize, look for changes/increases in vital signs, rapid changes in baseline mental status and behavior, increased confusion, assaultive behavior and self-stimulation at the site of pain.
6. Take a detailed history:
   - Assessment of pain intensity and characteristics
   - Full physical examination
   - Psychosocial assessment
   - Diagnostic evaluation based on signs and symptoms associated with the disease or syndrome causing the pain (such as arthritis and arthritis pain)
7. Identify what prompts the pain.
8. Identify what diminishes the pain.

Mneumonic "ABCDE":

A   Ask about pain regularly; Assess pain systematically.
B   Believe the patient and family in their reports of pain and what relieves it.
C   Choose pain control options appropriate for the patient, family, and setting.
D   Deliver interventions in a timely, logical, and coordinated fashion.
E   Empower patients and their families.
    Enable them to control their course to the greatest extent possible.

Adapted from Jacox, A., Carr, D.B., Payne, R., et al. *Management of Cancer Pain. Clinical Practice Guideline* No. 9. AHCPR Publication No. 94-0592. Rockville, MD. Agency for Health Care Policy and Research, US Dept. of Health and Human Services, Public Health Services, March 1994.

Appendix I

Pain Intensity Scales

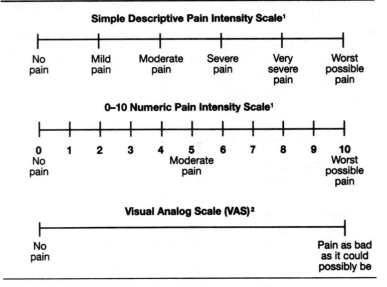

Simple Descriptive Pain Intensity Scale[1]

No pain | Mild pain | Moderate pain | Severe pain | Very severe pain | Worst possible pain

0–10 Numeric Pain Intensity Scale[1]

0 No pain 1 2 3 4 5 Moderate pain 6 7 8 9 10 Worst possible pain

Visual Analog Scale (VAS)[2]

No pain — Pain as bad as it could possibly be

[1] If used as a graphic rating scale, a 10 cm baseline is recommended.
[2] A 10-cm baseline is recommended for VAS scales.

Source: Acute Pain Management Guideline Panel, 1992.

Appendix J

Common Causes of Urinary Incontinence

- Delirium
- Infection
- Atrophic urethritis or vaginitis
- Sedative hypnotics
- Diuretics
- Anticholinergic agents (such as antihistamines, antidepressants, anti-spasmodics, anti-Parkinsonian agents)
- Alpha-adrenergic agents (antihypertensives, "cold" capsules)
- Calcium channel blockers
- Excessive urine production (from increased fluid intake, endocrine problems)
- Restricted mobility
- Stool impaction

Summarized from Urinary Incontinence Guideline Panel. *Urinary Incontinence in Adults: Quick Reference Guide for Clinicians.* AHCPR Pub. No. 92-0041. Rockville, MD: Agency for Health Care Policy and Research, Public Health Service, US Dept. of Health and Human Services, March 1992.

Glossary

Abduction movement away from the middle of the body.

Acrochordon a benign outgrowth of skin commonly found on axillae, eyelids, and neck; skin tag.

Acromegaly a condition of enlarged and elongated bones associated with hypersecretion of the human growth hormone.

Actinic keratoses a skin lesion associated with overexposure to sunlight; premalignant.

Activities of Daily Living (ADLs) activities necessary for living, including bathing, dressing, feeding, grooming, transferring, and toileting.

Adduction movement toward the middle of the body.

Adnexa Fallopian tubes, ovaries, and adjacent ligaments.

Advance directives specific directives made out while a person is competent and included in a legal document that outlines one's wishes in the event of debilitating illness.

Adventitious breath sounds abnormal additional breath sounds (wheezes, crackles, rhonchi).

Affective having to do with mood.

Ageusia loss of ability to taste.

Agraphia inability to write.

Air conduction sound traveling to the inner ear via air; air conduction takes longer than bone conduction.

Alexia inability to understand the meaning of a word/sentences.

Alveoli small packets of the lungs extending off the bronchioles.

Alzheimer's disease (AD) a chronic, progressive, irreversible form of dementia.

Andropause male stage of life similar to

menopause, occurring around 50 years of age, with reduction in male hormones (testosterone).

Anesthesia loss of sensation.

Angle of Louis manubriosternal juncture; where the manubrium and sternum meet.

Ankylosis joint stiffness and immobility.

Anorexia no appetite due to malaise, fever, medication, depression, or psychological disorders.

Aneurysm localized abnormal weakening or dilatation of a blood vessel, usually an artery.

Anus opening of the rectum.

Aorta begins at the upper portion of the left ventricle and extends as the major arterial network through the thorax, renal, abdominal, iliac, femoral, and tibial arteries.

Aphasia: expressive, receptive, and global

aphasia impaired ability to communicate.

expressive impaired ability to communicate verbally.

receptive impaired ability to understand.

global impaired ability to speak or understand.

Apical pulse pulse located at left midclavicular line at the 5th intercostal space, auscultated with a stethoscope; pulse heard at apex of the heart.

Apnea a period of breathing cessation lasting longer than 10 seconds.

Apraxia inability to actually verbalize a word that is thought of in the mind.

Aqueous humor liquid that passes through the posterior and anterior eye chambers.

Arcus senilis a white deposit of fat around the outer surface of the iris that does not normally interfere with vision.

Areola the circle of darker pigmentation around the nipple of each breast.

Arrhythmia irregular heart rhythm.

Arterial ulcers ulcers caused by arterial insufficiency; small, round, and smooth, often found on the foot and accompanied by pain and absent pulses (dorsalis pedis, posterior tibial, femoral, or popliteal).

Aspiration the inhaling of a substance other than air.

Assessment the first step in collecting subjective and objective data in the nursing process on which subsequent steps are based.

Astereognosis inability to identify objects by touch.

Atrioventricular node (AV node) controls electrical impulse of the heart, from atria to ventricles; 40 to 60 beats/minute is normal.

Atrium/atria upper two chambers of the heart.

Atrophic vaginitis inflammation of the vagina followed by menopause.

Auscultation investigation of the body by listening to its sounds.

Autonomic nervous system controls involuntary bodily functions.

Bartholin's cyst a cyst caused by blockage of fluid from Bartholin's glands, between the labia minora and hymenal ring.

Bell's Palsy facial paralysis on one side, from CN VII dysfunction; cause unknown.

Benign prostatic hyperplasia (BPH) increase in the number of cells in the prostate, often causing dysuria.

Blepharitis inflamed eyelids.

Blepharospasm a spasm of the orbicularis oculi muscle of the eye.

Blood pressure measure of the pressure from blood flowing in the large arteries.

Body transcendence versus body preoccupation one of three psychological developmental tasks

of old age described by Robert Peck: emphasis on cognitive and social skills to allow compensation for physical limitations that are part of everyday life with aging.

Bone conduction sound traveling through the inner ear via bone; air conduction takes longer than bone conduction.

Bone mineral density (BMD) x-rays for determining density of bones; aids in the diagnosis of osteoporosis.

Borborygmi loud bowel sounds.

Bradykinesia extreme slowness of movement.

Brachial pulse pulse palpated at the brachial artery.

Breast self-examination (BSE) systematic and regular inspection and palpation of breasts and surrounding tissues performed by an individual on self.

Bronchial tubes smaller tubes branching out from the bronchi.

Bronchophony sound heard when client says "99" or "1-2-3"; determines if lungs are filled with air, fluid, or solid.

Bronchovesicular sounds lung sound of moderate pitch and intensity heard at scapula and first or second intercostal spaces, equal on inspiration and expiration.

Bruits abnormal swishing sounds upon auscultating veins/vessels.

Cachexia muscle wasting.

Calorie a unit of heat measurement.

Candida vaginosa yeast cells that in excess create a white drainage and itching in the vaginal area.

Canker sore red sore found in mouth or on lips.

Capillary refill test pinching and blanching the finger nail bed and assessing the seconds it takes color to return.

Cardiac cycle excitation of the heart allowing for the contraction and blood flow through the body.

Carotid pulse pulse felt at the carotid artery.

Carpal tunnel syndrome numbness in hand, wrist, and arm due to overuse and trauma to the hand muscles.

Cataract opacity (cloudiness) of the eye's lens.

Central axillary nodes lymph nodes found in the axillae.

Central nervous system brain and spinal cord.

Cerebral vascular accident (CVA, stroke) the obstruction of the blood and oxygen supply to a segment of the brain caused by a thrombus, an embolus, or bleeding.

Cerumen ear wax.

Cervical smear obtaining a lab specimen of the outer tissue at the inferior aspect of the uterus.

Chancre red, round ulcer with raised edges and an indurated center.

Chandler's sign tenderness of the cervix on palpation.

Cheyne-Stokes breathing cyclical periods of breathing paired with no breathing.

Chief complaint the main problem for which a person seeks health care.

Chlamydia a bacteria that grows intracellularly and causes various lung and genital infections.

Circumlocution unable to answer a question/topic; "circling around" a topic.

Clicks and gurgles sounds heard in the abdomen connoting peristalsis (movement of food and gastric juices through the digestive tract).

Clitoris located at the superior aspect of the vulva between the labia minora; contains erectile tissue with numerous nerve endings.

Cognition the mental capacity characterized by recognition, memory, processing, learning, and judgment.

Colostomy surgical opening of the colon to the external abdomen.

Complete health history detailed past and present health history of a client.

Confabulation a "making up" of answers when memory fails.

Conjunctivitis inflammation of the conjunctiva of the eye due to infection or trauma.

Cooper's ligaments ligaments that provide support to breast tissue; extend vertically through the fascia to inner skin layer through the breast.

Coronary arteries the two major arteries, left and right, which feed blood to the myocardium.

Cortical bone outer layer of bone.

Costal angle angle where the costal margins meet at the sternum.

Crackles a snapping sound heard on lung auscultation in a person who has atelectasis or other situations of alveolar closure. Formerly called rales. A similar sound can be obtained by twisting and rubbing your hair right behind the ear.

Cranial nerves the twelve pairs of nerves emanating from the brain.

Crepitus a grating sound as in bone against bone.

Crohn's disease chronic inflammation of the bowel.

Cullen's sign bluish color around umbilicus suggesting peritoneal bleeding.

Cuticle (nail) tissue between the nail bed and nail.

Cystocele anterior vaginal wall protrusion.

Deep tendon reflexes (DTR) reflexes deep within the tendons, tested to assess central nervous system function.

Deep vein thrombosis (DVT) a clot or thrombus occurring in the veins, usually in a leg.

Degenerative joint disease (DJD) wearing away at the joints resulting in stiffness and decreased range of motion.

Dehydration excessive loss of water from body tissues.

Delirium a rapid-onset state of confusion, disorientation, delusions, and sometimes hallucinations that is usually reversible with prompt appropriate treatment.

Dementia a slow-onset, irreversible state of cognitive defects that can be the result of a medical condition or disease (such as Alzheimer's), substance reaction (such as long-term alcoholism), or a combination of these factors.

Depression various degrees of feeling sad, helpless, hopeless, and perhaps suicidal.

Dermis the second layer of skin.

Developmental task a growth responsibility that occurs at a particular time in life.

Diaphoresis excessive perspiration.

Dorsalis pedis pulse pulse palpated at the top of the foot between the first and second toes.

Dyesthesia misinterpretation of a stimulus, such as feeling a sharp stimulus as tingling.

Dysarthria lack of muscular control in mouth, face, neck, throat, or brain needed to speak.

Dyspareunia difficult, painful intercourse.

Dysphagia difficulty in swallowing.

Dysphasia speech impairment due to brain dysfunction.

Dysphonia inability to make sounds of a word due to disease of the larynx.

Dyspnea labored or difficult breathing.

Dysuria difficulty urinating

Ecchymosis "black-and-blue" mark; red-purple discoloration/bruise.

Eccrine sweat glands.

Ectropion eversion of the eyelids.

Edema swelling; fluid excess.

Edentulous being without natural teeth.

Ego differentiation versus work and role preoccupation one of three psychological developmental tasks of old age described by Robert Peck: the development of valued alternatives in addition to one's work-role, acting to reaffirm self-worth.

Ego integrity versus despair the eighth stage of development described by Eric Erikson as self-acceptance (ego integrity) versus dissatisfaction with life (despair).

Ego transcendence versus ego preoccupation one of three psychological developmental tasks of old age described by Robert Peck: development of the ability to devote energies to the welfare of future generations without preoccupation with one's own death.

Egophony sound produced when client says "ee;" used to assess presence of air, fluid, or solid in the lungs.

Elastosis breakdown of connective tissue protein, elastin.

Elder mistreatment acts of commission (intentional infliction of harm) or acts of omission (harm occurring through neglect) taken by a caregiver.

Elite older adult person 85 years or older.

Enterostomal therapy nurse (ETN) a nurse that specializes in ostomy care.

Entropion eyelids that turn in causing the possibility of infection in the eye.

Epidermis outer layer of skin.

Episodic health history a specific, problem-generated client history, usually narrow and pertinent to the issue at hand.

Erythema redness of the skin.

Estrogen replacement therapy (ERT) hormone therapy given after menopause when the natural production of estrogen decreases.

Evaluation the final step of the nursing process that measures the client's degree of goal achievement.

Exophthalmos excessive protrusion of the eye.

External rotation turning outward.

Extrapyramidal outside the tracts of the central nervous system; emanates from the cortical and subcortical motor area structures of the brain.

Failure to Thrive (FTT) in the absence of physiological etiology, the syndrome of overall decline, weight loss, and hopelessness thought to be caused by psychological deprivation.

Fall Efficacy Scale (FES) a self-appraisal instrument to assess fall risk.

Femoral pulse the pulse palpated at the femoral artery.

Food Guide Pyramid guideline to improve food choices based on low-fat, high-fiber intake.

Forward flexion bending limb, body, or joint forward.

Fovea centralis middle of the macula that allows for sharpness of sight.

Functional status ability of a person to carry out ADLs, IADLs, and social activities.

Gastroesophogeal reflex disorder (GERD) persistent reflux of the stomach contents into the esophagus.

Genogram a diagrammatic display of a person's family health history.

Genitalia male and female reproductive organs.

Gerontology an interdisciplinary study of the process of aging.

Gerontological nursing the holistic nursing care of sick and well older adults.

Gingivitis inflammation of the gums.

Glasgow Coma Scale widely used scale for grading neurological response.

Glaucoma an eye disease characterized by increased intraocular pressure; it can cause blindness without treatment.

Goiter enlarged thyroid.

Gonorrhea a sexually transmitted disease caused by the bacteria *Neissera gonorrhoeae*.

Graves' Disease disease of hyperthyroidism, with weight loss, heat intolerance, and eye and dermal involvement.

Gynecomastia collection of adipose tissue at the site of male breast tissue.

Heaves lifting of the cardiac area due to increased workload on the heart.

Heberden's nodes node thickening and enlargement at the distal phalanges of the fingers.

Hemorrhoids swelling of the hemorrhoidal veins in the rectum resulting in difficulty having a bowel movement.

Hepatic pertaining to the liver.

Herpes simplex caused by the virus of same name and resulting in eruption of vesicles in the oral area.

Hiatal hernia protrusion of a portion of the stomach through the diaphragm.

Hirschberg test symmetrical reflection of light off the cornea.

Hirsutism excessive body hair growth.

Hierarchy of needs a hierarchical framework consisting of five levels developed by Abraham Maslow to explain a person's level of functioning.

Homan's sign quick dorsiflexion of the foot resulting in pain (suggests venous thrombosis in the calf) or no pain.

Hordeolum a sty located in the eyelid.

Hormone replacement therapy (HRT) the use of hormones such as estrogen, progesterone, and testosterone (in small amounts) to supplement and eventually replace the natural ones that decline with menopause. Estrogen HRT is believed to prevent osteoporosis and reduce the incidence of heart disease in postmenopausal women.

Hydrocele the collection of fluid, especially in a cavity (such as the tunica vaginalis of the testis).

Hyperesthesia excessive sensitivity to touch.

Hyperextension extreme extension.

Hyperthyroidism the thyroid's over-secretion of thyroxine.

Hypoesthesia reduced sense of touch.

Hypogeusia reduction in the ability to taste.

Hypothalamus controls metabolic functions, fluid balance, body temperature, and hormonal balance.

Hypothyroidism reduced thyroid secretion requiring hormone replacement therapy.

Iatrogenic complication or disease caused by medical treatment and/or health care providers.

Ileostomy surgical opening and fecal drainage from the abdominal wall at the ileum.

Implementation portion of the nursing process focused on nursing interventions or approaches to facilitate the client's goal accomplishment.

Infraclavicular nodes lymph nodes located at the cavities of the clavicles.

Inorgasmia inability to experience an orgasm.

Isolated systolic hypertension a specific type of high blood pressure.

Inspection the skill of detailed and specific observation to assess an individual's health.

Instrumental Activities of Daily Living (IADL) managing money, shopping, housekeeping, preparing meals, and taking medications correctly.

Interdisciplinary approach/care care of geriatric patients requiring complex systems that involve numerous services and therapies. It is usually made up of health care providers (physicians, nurses, social workers, dietitians, psychologists, and others in the health care field).

Internal rotation turning inward.

Intervention a purposeful nursing action focused at a positive client outcome.

IOP (intraocular pressure) pressure within the eye, not related to blood pressure.

Iris "eye color" of the eye; front portion of the uveal tract of the eye.

Irritable bowel disease pain and cramping in the small and large intestines; constipation alternating with diarrhea; triggered by anxiety and dietary habits.

Jugular vein pressure (JVP) pressure in the jugular vein observed and measured with the client in a sitting position; a good indicator of central venous pressure.

Kegel exercises contracting exercises of the perineum to help treat urinary incontinence.

Korotkoff sounds alteration in sounds as blood pressure cuff inflates around the arm.

Kussmaul's breathing increase in rate and depth of respiration, as in diabetic ketoacidosis.

Kyphosis "humpback"; convexation of the spine.

Lacrimal gland gland in the eye that secretes tears.

Lateral nodes lymph nodes located alongside body landmarks.

Left ventricular hypertrophy (LVH) enlargement of the left ventricle of the heart.

Leukoplakia white patches on tongue or cheeks.

Level of consciousness (LOC) degree to which an individual manifests alertness; ranges from alert to comatose.

Life review systematically evaluating one's successes and failures in life, with professional help, to resolve conflicts and prepare for death. Butler's concept that states that it is the awareness of one's own death that elicits an evaluation of one's life and how one has lived it.

Lipoma fatty tumor.

Lithotomy position supine with knees bent.

Low-density lipids (LDL) cholesterol that contributes to blockage of arteries and cardiovascular disease.

Lungs the two spongy organs in the thoracic cavity used for breathing.

Lymph nodes alkaline fluid-filled nodal network throughout the body cavities used to cleanse tissues and fight infection.

Malnutrition inadequate amount and quality of food intake.

Manubrium top of sternum.

Mastectomy removal of breast or breast tissue.

McBurney's point a point in the right lower quadrant of the abdomen situated in the area of the appendix.

Menopause cessation of menses in women in their late 40s to mid-50s due mainly to decreased estrogen production.

Mental health feelings of personal wellness and successful adaptation to the outside world.

Miotic pupillary contraction.

Mitral valve valve between left atrium and left ventricle.

Mononucleosis caused by Epstein-Barr or other virus with increase in mononuclear leukocytes characterized by flu symptoms.

Murmur abnormal blowing, hissing, or swishing sounds of the heart.

Mutual goal-setting establishing a client's health care goals involving both client and health care team.

Mydriatic causing pupillary dilation.

Myopia able to see only a short distance due to faulty lens refraction.

Myxedema swelling, specific to thyroid dysfunction.

Nail root proximal part of the nail.

Nailbed nail portion of the finger or toe.

Normal aging aging-related changes that occur in the absence of disease.

Nursing diagnosis the client problem, as identified using specific taxonomy.

Nutrition Screening Initiative (NSI) government, American Dietetic Association, and American Academy of Family Physicians' joint effort in the early 1990s to promote better nutrition in the older adult population.

Nystagmus involuntary movements of the eye.

Occipital area back of head.

Occupational therapist professional trained in facilitating self-care, work skills, and leisure activities to enhance client independence.

Olecranon process bony parts of the elbow.

Ophthalmologist physician specializing in eye diseases.

Ophthalmoscope instrument used to inspect and examine the eye.

Optometrist professional who treats visual abnormalities as determined per state regulation. Scope of practice is not as expansive as that of the ophthalmologist.

Orientation awareness of person, place, and time in reality.

Orthopnea a respiratory symptom in which the person breathes most comfortably when in an upright position.

Orthostatic hypotension *see* postural hypotension.

Osteoarthritis degeneration of joints related to wear and tear.

Osteomyelitis bone infection.

Osteoporosis weakening and hollowing (decrease in bone mass) of the bones.

Otoscope instrument used to examine the ear.

Outcome consequence of interventions.

Paget's disease inflammation of bones and a thickening and softening of bones; sometimes a bowing of legs.

Pain assessment assessment that includes measures of pain intensity and pain experience, a combination that is important in evaluating chronic pain.

Pain, chronic pain that extends past the normally expected time of healing. Pain that extends 3 months is commonly accepted as chronic within a clinical context, whereas 6 months is preferred for research purposes.

Palpation understanding the body through deep and light touch.

Papanicolaou test a diagnostic test of the cervix to determine abnormal conditions such as cancer.

Papilloma superficial tumor.

Paranoid suspicious thoughts and delusions characterized by intense feelings of persecution and threatening hallucinations.

Parasympathetic nervous system includes cranial and sacral nerves.

Paresthesia numbness or tingling; an abnormal sensation.

Parietal area part of brain controlling somatic and sensory feelings.

Parkinson's disease a neurological deficiency of dopamine, which results in a variety of symptoms, primarily tremor, muscle rigidity, and slow movement.

Paroxysmal nocturnal dyspnea (PND) severe respiratory distress at night while sleeping flat, relieved by sitting up, and due to left side heart failure.

Pathological aging age-related changes that are primarily a function of underlying disease states and are therefore not normal.

Pathological reflexes abnormal reflexes.

Pectoral nodes lymph nodes surrounding the pectoral area.

Peptic ulcer disease stomach, duodenal, or jejunal ulcer.

Percussion tapping parts of the body to determine abnormal versus normal conditions by sounds.

Pericardial friction rub sound heard during inspiration caused by an inflamed pericardium.

Perineum external area between vulva and anus, or scrotum and anus.

Periodontal disease disease of the gums and alveolar bones of the mouth. The common cause of tooth loss in older people. Can be prevented with proper care.

Peripheral nervous system cranial and spinal nerves.

Peritoneum lining of the abdominal cavity.

Periungual tissue tissue around the nail.

Pharmacokinetics the absorption, distribution, metabolism, and excretion of drugs in the body.

Physical therapist professional who focuses on rehabilitation and restoration of function emphasizing muscles and bones.

Planning aspect of nursing process that focuses on planning for actual care.

Plantar reflex foot reflex.

Pleural friction rub inflammation of the pleura resulting in a grating sound upon auscultation.

Polypharmacy the administration of multiple prescription and nonprescription medications simultaneously; often seen with older persons resulting in increased adverse effects.

Popliteal pulse pulse located behind knees.

Posterior tibial pulse pulse located at back of foot adjacent to Achilles tendon.

Postural hypotension a condition in which the blood pressure falls when changing to an upright position, resulting in dizziness or fainting.

Precordium term connoting frontal area over heart and thorax.

Presbycusis decreased ability to hear as one ages.

Presbyopia increased farsightedness (impaired near vision) in later middle age.

Pressure ulcer sore created mainly by pressure constricting blood flow to an area.

Pronator drift unilateral drift in one arm when client closes eyes and holds arms out, due to neurological problem such as stroke.

Prostate specific antigen (PSA) a screening blood test that indicates an abnormal condition of the prostate, especially cancer.

Pruritis excessive itching.

Psychotropics mood-altering drugs.

Pterygium yellow thickening of the conjunctiva.

Ptosis drooping eyelid.

Pulmonic area auscultated at second intercostal space left of the sternum.

Pulsation rhythmic beating or throbbing.

Pulse rhythmic movement of blood flow through arteries.

Pulse deficit when radial pulse is less than apical pulse.

Pulse oximetry indirect measurement of oxygenation via a sensor on the outside of the body: often on ear lobe or finger.

Quality of life what the individual determines is quality relative to her or his life.

Radial pulse pulse located at the wrist at the base of the thumb.

Rales *see* crackles.

Range of motion (ROM) the range of movement of a joint; the "north-south-east-west" movement of limbs; may be active (self-movement) or passive (movement of a limb by another).

Rate the numerical counting or speed of something such as heart beats per minute.

Reminiscence therapy thinking and talking about mostly pleasant memories from the past.

Respiration inhale-exhale breathing cycle.

Rectocele protrusion through the vagina of the posterior vaginal wall.

Red reflex shining light from the ophthalmoscope into the pupil onto the retina, which should reflect a light reflection.

Registered Dietician (R.D.) the health professional whose expertise is in nutrition.

Required Dietary Allowances (RDA) national recommendations for the daily intake of certain vitamins and minerals by age groups.

Review of systems (ROS) client's subjective response to body system questions, which must be confirmed through examination and other data.

Rhythm regularity in sound or movement, such as in a beating heart or breathing.

Ringworm skin infection caused by various fungi, noted by a red-ringed patch of vesicles that itch.

Rinne test use of a tuning fork to test for bone versus air conduction through the ear canal.

Scapula flat, triangular bone at the posterior shoulders.

Scoliosis curvature of the spine, laterally.

Sebaceous glands glands that secrete sebum, a fatty oil.

Seborrhea dandruff.

Seborrheic keratosis benign skin tumor.

Sebum the body's natural oil.

Self-care ability to meet one's own daily needs.

Self-care deficit various degrees of inability to care for self.

Self-esteem individual's sense of self-worth.

Self-neglect inability to provide self-care to meet basic needs.

Senescence the process of aging; the biological, physiological, sociological, and psychological changes that accompany the aging process.

Sensory impairment decrease in one or more of the five senses (sight, hearing, taste, smell, touch).

Sexually transmitted diseases (STDs) diseases transmitted through oral/genital contact.

Sinoatrial node (SA node) nerves in the heart that initiate electrical activity needed for cardiac muscle contraction.

Sleep apnea cessation of respiration during sleep lasting longer than 10 seconds.

Snellen chart chart used to test vision; ranges from small to large letters.

Social roles the activities, rights, and responsibilities that accompany a particular position in society.

Social skills interactional techniques required for integration into society.

Social support a person, agency, or organization from which one receives individual assistance, encouragement, and comfort when needed.

Speculum instrument used to view body cavity, such as bivalve speculum to view the vagina.

Speech/language pathologist a professional who specializes in diagnosis and treatment of speech and language abnormalities.

Spermatocele tumor located in the epididymis.

Spinal processes bony protrusions from the vertebrae of the spine.

Spiritual well-being the affirmation of life in a relationship with a God, self, community, and environment that nurtures and celebrates wholeness.

Spirituality belief in a greater life form and existence.

Stereognosis identification of objects by touch.

Sternocleidomastoid muscle at the inner part of the clavicle.

Sternum flat bone dividing the anterior thorax.

Subcutaneous tissue tissue directly beneath the epidermis.

Subluxation partial dislocation of a bone.

Subscapular nodes lymph nodes located in the cavity below the shoulder blades.

Sundown syndrome increased degree of confusion and disorientation that occurs in older persons with dementia in the late afternoon or early evening.

Sunrise syndrome decreased cognitive functioning early in the morning.

Superficial reflexes reflexes related to surface nerves.

Supraclavicular nodes lymph nodes located above the clavicles.

Sympathetic nervous system starts from thoracic and lumbar spine; when stimulated, increases heart rate, dilates pupils, and increases epinephrine and norepinephrine in response to stressors.

Tactile fremitus vibrations felt when hands are placed on client's chest.

Tail of Spence upper outer part of the chest, which extends into the axilla.

Tardive dyskinesia abnormal movements of the tongue, neck, fingers, trunk, and legs caused by some antipsychotic medications.

Telangiectasia lesion consisting of small blood vessels.

Temperature body heat measured in Fahrenheit or Celsius units.

Temporal area below frontal lobe of brain; controls some auditory functions.

Temporal pulse pulse located at temple.

Temporomandibular joint (TMJ) between mandible and temporal bones; if inflamed or stiff, creates pain and clicking in the jaw area.

Testicular torsion a twisting or strangulation of the testes causing circulatory blockage; emergency surgery is required.

Thalamus mediates sensory stimuli, pain, temperature, and aspects of touch.

Thomas test knee to chest movement while supine; remaining leg should stay flat on the examination table.

Thorax chest cavity.

Thrills quivering felt from a cardiac murmur.

Tinetti Balance and Gait Evaluation a seventeen-item scored instrument used to assess gait plus balance; the lower the score, the greater the likelihood of imbalance.

Tonometry measures intraocular pressure to detect glaucoma.

Torticollis neck deformity, with head tilted to one side.

Trabecular bone woven, meshed tissue found inside the bones.

Trachea tubular structure from larynx to bronchi.

Tragus protrusion at the external anterior ear.

Transient ischemic attack (TIA) a stroke, which comes and goes (is transient); symptoms of a stroke that usually last 20 minutes to 24 hours and can be a predictor of a major stroke.

Tricuspid valve heart valve between the right atrium and right ventricle.

Turgor tautness; tension of the skin often referred to as skin turgor.

Tympany hollow sound, like that made by beating on a drum.

Unna boot layered gauze dressing of lower extremities used in treatment of venous leg ulcers.

Urethral meatus opening of the bladder as it exits the body.

Urinary tract infection (UTI) bacterial infection of the bladder, ureter, and/or kidneys.

Uvula soft structure hanging at the soft palate in the back of the throat.

Vaginal introitus entrance into the vagina.

Venous hum continuous hum heard in veins; may suggest anemia.

Venous ulcers sores usually found on the lower legs caused by venous insufficiency stasis.

Ventricle two lower chambers of the heart; left chamber pumps blood to the aorta and out to the body; right chamber pumps blood to the pulmonary artery and lungs.

Vertebra prominens 7th cervical vertebra.

Vertigo dizziness; feeling of motion and unbalance of equilibrium.

Vesicular sounds soft, smooth sounds heard in normal lungs.

Vital signs temperature, pulse, respiration, blood pressure, and degree of comfort/pain.

Weber test tests for nerve or conductive hearing loss.

Wheezes abnormal, high-pitched whistling breath sounds.

Xanthelasma nodule found on eyelids near inner canthus.

Xerophthalmia a sequence of abnormalities of increasing severity in the conjunctiva and cornea of the eye caused by vitamin A deficiency. Rare in the United States but common in Southeast Asia and parts of Africa and South America.

Xerosis excessively dry skin.

Xiphoid process protrusion at lower part of sternum; calcifies as people age.

Index